LEADERSHIP FOR GREAT CUSTOMER SERVICE

Satisfied Patients,
Satisfied Employees

LEADERSHIP FOR GREAT CUSTOMER SERVICE

Satisfied Patients,

Satisfied Employees

Thom A. Mayer

Robert J. Cates

ACHE Management Series

Health Administration Press

Your board, staff, or clients may also benefit from this book's insight. For more information on quantity discounts, contact the Health Administration Press Marketing Manager at (312) 424-9470.

October 2013 Reprinting

Library of Congress Cataloging-in-Publication Data

Mayer, Thom A.
    Leadership for great customer service: satisfied patients, satisfied employees / Thom Mayer & Robert J. Cates.
        p. cm.
    Includes bibliographical references.
    ISBN 1-56793-228-2 (alk. paper)
      1. Patient satisfaction. 2. Medical personnel and patient. 3. Medical care—Quality control. I. Cates, Robert J. II. Title.

R727.3.M385 2004
362.11′068′8—dc22

                                       2004049129

The paper used in this publication meets the minimum requirements of American National Standard for Information Sciences—Permanence of Paper for Printed Library Materials, ANSI Z39.48-1984. ♾™

Acquisitions manager: Janet Davis; Project manager: Cami Cacciatore; Layout editor: Amanda Karvelaitis; Cover designer: Trisha Lartz

Health Administration Press
A division of the Foundation of the
   American College of Healthcare Executives
1 North Franklin Street, Suite 1700
Chicago, IL 60606-4425
(312) 424-2800

To my beautiful and brilliant wife, Maureen; our kind, generous, and thoughtful sons, Josh, Kevin and Gregory; and to my father, affectionately known to everyone as Grandpa Jim. Their love and support have sustained me in this and all other work.

— *Thom A. Mayer, M.D.*

To my wife, Kim; my children, Beth, Rob and Jill; my mother, Phyllis; and my sister, Debbie, in appreciation of your love and support.

— *Robert J. Cates, M.D.*

In memory of a
trusted colleague and dear friend,
Martin Gottlieb.

Contents

Foreword

IN THE MADNESS of the modern world of healthcare, write Doctors Thom Mayer and Robert Cates in *Leadership for Great Customer Service,* technical excellence is a necessary but insufficient condition for institutional survival. The missing link, they argue persuasively (and based on an impressive body of research and "clinical practice" with service initiatives), is a strategic and cultural commitment to excellent customer service.

I honestly can't remember when I've seen so much of so much importance crammed into a short book. The authors do an excellent job of making the case for customer service excellence in acute care institutions. They go on to provide assistance in making the case with staffs. Then they lay out, with surpassing clarity, the process for embedding a service excellence culture in a medical institution. Finally, they devote the last third of the book to the details of program implementation, down to the important role of body language in patient-staff interactions. They do all of this in a little over a hundred pages, which are almost breezy (while serious) and jargon free, though written specifically for the healthcare professional. All in all, this is a masterful effort, and one that is long overdue.

Without (I hope) giving away the punch line, let me share in summary form my highlights tape:

- Customer-service initiatives don't work unless they make the job easier for staff. Hint: They can!
- It takes a revolution. "All this" is more than a program, it's a *way of life*, a cultural about-face, lived strategically and in the grubby moment-to-moment details.
- There are A-team players and B-team players. B-team players are probably in the wrong job, and one at any level can destroy an entire shift. Deal with it: Work assiduously on improvement, and dump those who in the end don't/can't/won't get it.
- There is an enormous difference between a patient and a customer. Customers are vertical. Patients are horizontal. The majority of throughput is customers, and customers require a very different approach than patients. (The discussion of working with staff on identifying biases and clarifying definitions is worth the price of admission alone.)
- The service diagnosis is as important as the clinical diagnosis. And the approach to the two diagnoses is very different.
- Even in the lofty atmosphere of acute care medicine, one can, on occasion, turn an angry customer-patient into a friend and fan with a $25 gift certificate to Outback Steakhouse.
- Service excellence ultimately depends on the management of *moments of truth*, a collection of usually small incidents involving staff-patient interaction. These can be clearly identified, and responses can be meticulously scripted.
- Never cross your arms while talking to a patient-customer.

And so on.

In fact, a lot of this is right out of the Disney-Nordstrom playbook (though one of the authors had a single, nasty experience with Nordstrom—and never went back). Mayer and Cates acknowledge their debt to such exemplary institutions but point out that healthcare professionals have great difficulty (understatement, in my experience) analogizing from the pixie-dust world of Disney to the life-and-death world of emergency services. Make no mistake, while the lessons here are indeed universal, they come from healthcare research and program implementation, use healthcare cases, are couched in healthcare language, and deal with healthcare "objections."

Leadership for Great Customer Service is laserlike in its aim. It is not a screed on lousy service. It is not an Rx for healthcare in general. It is a terse, complete, focused, readable, at times amusing guide to addressing perhaps the number one opportunity for any acute care institution to win customer affection while making the working environment and staff's life more attractive simultaneously. Not a bad deal!

—Tom Peters
Lenox, Massachusetts

Acknowledgments

NO BOOK IS ever the sole product of the authors themselves. Instead, any book reflects the complex interactions of the many, many people with whom the authors have interacted to produce the thoughts reflected in their book. In our case, this fact is expanded exponentially by the literally thousands of participants in our Survival Skills courses with whom we have interacted over a ten year period to refine these concepts.

Our first debt is to those who attended our courses. Our colleagues at BestPractices, Inc. (formerly Emergency Physicians of Northern Virginia, Ltd.) and Inova Fairfax Hospital have been supportive of our work and exemplify daily the best in healthcare customer service. The emergency department nurses with whom we have worked at the Inova Health System, Potomac Hospital, and many other facilities have enriched our lives beyond measure and have contributed to many of the thoughts and strategies reflected in this book.

The members of the Physician Leadership Team at BestPractices, Inc. are as fine a team of healthcare leaders as any in the nation, and their thoughts have contributed to the development of the Survival Skills concept. These individuals include doctors Michael Altieri, Raul

Armengol, Damian Banaszak, Glenn Druckenbrod, Luis Eljaiek, Jr., Keith Ghezzi, Dan Hanfling, William Hauda, John Howell, Kathleen Kelly, Kathryn Kenders, Maybelle Kou, John Maguire, Mary Ann McLaurin, Judy Mechanick, Peter Paganussi, Denis Pauze, Rick Place, and Scott Weir; and Rick Bishow, PA-C.

We have had the good fortune to work with some of the finest healthcare administrators in the country, all of whom have been supportive of our commitment to customer service, including J. Knox Singleton, Jolene Tornabeni, Toni Ardabell, Steven Brown, Mary Jane Mastorovich, Edward Eroe, Charles Barnett, William Flannagan, Jr., William Moss, Joan Miles, Tom Corder, and Richard Stull. Without their support, the team nature of Survival Skills training could not have developed in the compelling fashion it has.

Joy Sparks-Gaviria was patient and painstakingly attentive to every detail in the creation and submission of this manuscript. Simply stated, the book could not have been completed without her excellent work. Her efforts are also appreciated during the scheduling of the Survival Skills training sessions, where she is always referred to as "a joy to work with."

In addition, the entire support staff at BestPractices, Inc., led by Kaye Wear and Kristi Hurst, participated in various ways in the development of this work.

Many thanks to Tom Peters, both for contributing his generous and thoughtful foreword to this book and for his friendship and mentoring over the years. To have the guidance of such an internationally recognized thought leader is fortune beyond belief.

The chair of BestPractices, Inc.'s board of directors, Russ Ramsey, has taught us a great deal about the importance of customer service, as well as many other aspects of the application of business principles to healthcare.

For their patience with a decade of hard work, long hours, and travel to every corner of the country, I (Thom) thank my wonderful wife, Maureen, and our sons, Josh, Kevin, and Gregory. Without their patience, understanding, and forbearance, neither the Survival Skills concept nor this book would have happened.

For her unwavering support, abundant wisdom, and uncommon common sense, I (Bob) thank my wife, Kim, and my three children, Beth, Rob, and Jill, who continually teach me.

Audrey Kaufman and Janet Davis at Health Administration Press are experienced, insightful, and highly professional acquisitions editors who improved both the content and the presentation of this work. No author could ask for better assistance. Cami Cacciatore's editing was as precise as a surgeon's knife and is greatly appreciated.

To our friend and colleague Dr. Irwin Press goes our deepest respect and admiration for the many conversations we have had over the years regarding patient satisfaction and how best to attain it.

Joan Kyes, RN, was an essential part of the birth of the Survival Skills concept. Her insights on stress, change management, and human behavior are critical parts of the development of this book and the course on which it was based. Her friendship, guidance, and humor have enriched not only this book but our lives as well.

If we have neglected to mention the many others who have contributed to our lives and our thinking about customer service, it is only because of space limitations and does not reflect the depth of our gratitude and appreciation.

Introduction

THIS BOOK GREW out of a decade of experience in researching and teaching the application of the art of customer service to the science of clinical medicine. Like many ideas, the concept of healthcare customer service is a simple one, yet excruciatingly difficult to execute; therefore, we focused our efforts on execution. In 1994, as we researched excellence in customer service, we found very few training programs designed to apply customer service to healthcare. Even those that existed suffered either from the "argument from authority" flaw ("Do it because the boss says so!") or from a lack of pragmatic approaches to applying service skills in the healthcare arena. Faced with this problem—and with a clear need to significantly improve the customer service we offered in our institution—we created a training course called Survival Skills designed to systematically teach service excellence skills to our staff.

We felt several requirements were necessary to make such a course successful. First, we knew that healthcare workers were used to systematic, protocol-oriented approaches to clinical care. The Advanced Cardiac Life Support (ACLS), the Advanced Pediatric Life Support (APLS), and the Advanced Trauma Life Support (ATLS) courses were all examples of how clearly delineated course material and skills could be communicated to help improve the care of the patients. Basically, we set out to create the ACLS, APLS, ATLS course for customer service in healthcare. Second, like any change effort, we felt that we needed to appeal to intrinsic rather than extrinsic motivation to sustain a successful change management effort—in this case a transformation to service excellence in healthcare. Therefore, we needed to show the staff that developing service excellence skills was not only in our patients' best interest but in their own interest as well. Third, it was our belief that the course had to be taught by active clinicians involved in the care of the patient. During an early course we taught at an academic medical center in New York, one of the nurses in the audience told us after the course, "You guys were really good! But if you had been from Macy's, we would have eaten you alive!" Her insight was important: Healthcare professionals paid attention to us because they knew we took care of patients, but if we had been from a different industry and had tried to exhort them to provide better customer service, they would have never paid attention to us, much less the principles we espoused. Finally, we knew that the material had to be extremely practical, with clear advice on how to apply it to the patients.

Did it work? The answer is an enthusiastic "Yes!" Not only did our customer service scores improve dramatically following the implementation of the Survival Skills concept but they have stayed at industry-leading levels since that time and have continued to improve. Moreover, the Survivals Skills course has been taught to hundreds of hospitals with thousands of participants, resulting in dramatic improvements in their customer service ratings as well. Our physician management and leadership company, which provides emergency department and other hospital-based physicians for hospitals and healthcare systems, is committed to

The **SCIENCE** of Clinical Excellence
The **ART** of Customer Service
The **BUSINESS** of Execution

Creating the **FUTURE** of Healthcare

So customer service excellence is one of the three legs of our business strategy—and clearly one of the most important. This book is intended to share the insights we have gained from over 25 years of experience in providing clinical care, healthcare leadership, and training in customer service. While the book is carefully researched, it is intended to be used as a practical resource in understanding and applying customer service to healthcare, and it includes stories, quotations, training exercises, and the use of examples throughout. The "More on This" section at the end of each chapter offers an annotated bibliography of the writings that we most respect and admire on the topics.

Chapter 1 sets the stage for the transformation to a culture of customer service by emphasizing that all fundamental, meaningful, and lasting change is intrinsically rather than extrinsically motivated. The chapter illustrates ways to demonstrate both the importance of the intrinsic nature of change in customer service and how to deal with those who create a negative effect in your organization.

Chapter 2 addresses the difficult question, "Are those we care for in healthcare patients or customers?" by offering three clinical scenarios to demonstrate that healthcare providers ask this question (whether consciously or subconsciously) with nearly every clinical interaction. It is up to us as healthcare leaders to make sure our staffs know that we should treat the customer component with service skills (which are delineated in Chapters 3 through 6) and the patient component with technical skills.

The third chapter introduces the first Survival Skill: Making the Customer Service Diagnosis and Offering the Right Treatment. It builds on the insight from the previous chapter that we must recognize that those we care for are both patients and customers and therefore require both service and technical excellence skills. The importance of effective communication and the use of scripting are also addressed in this chapter.

Chapter 4 discusses the second Survival Skill: Negotiating Agreement and Resolution of Expectations. The dissonance between the patient/customer's expectations and those of your healthcare staff can often be dramatic and must be addressed through negotiation. Negotiation is a critically important skill in healthcare, since you negotiate constantly, not just with your patients/customers but with your staff as well. We also present three negotiation steps and six tools (and examples of each).

Chapter 5 presents the third Survival Skill: Creating Moments of Truth. After reviewing the "moments of truth" concept, we illustrate that healthcare is fundamentally a personal service business, where the people performing the service are the company, at least from the patient/customer's perspective. Multiple strategies for meaningfully and reliably creating moments of truth are presented, as well as the concept of rewarding service champions, celebrating success, and promoting for service excellence. The chapter ends with suggestions on how to help your staff recognize that they are truly heroes and that they provide a critically important service to those most in need of care and compassion.

The final chapter is a practical survey of how to put these Survival Skills concepts to work in your institution. Like any good user's manual it gives pragmatic advice on how to apply these principles with your leadership and management team.

In some ways it is unfortunate and regrettable that there is a need for a practical book on customer service. After decades of experience in healthcare leadership, it is in many respects surprising that so little useful, practical, and uniform means of training for customer service exist. Yet the fact remains that many healthcare institutions have never quite figured out how to make customer service real throughout the organization. Our experience has been that our Survival Skills approach works dramatically, as long as you, the healthcare leader, remain unceasingly committed to continuing to improve service excellence using the practical approaches we have outlined in the book. The number one reason to get customer service right is to make your job easier.

Our fondest expectation is that this book, and the principles that it espouses, makes the job easier for you as a healthcare leader and for those you guide toward better service excellence at your institution.

We hope you find something worthwhile in these pages. Please steal our work. Use our stories and examples. Nothing could please us more than knowing you and your staff found some small part of this worth sharing with those who care for others. We believe these are Survival Skills—skills your staff will need to survive in the busy milieu of healthcare. Please feel free to contact us by telephone, mail, or e-mail if there is anything we can do to help. And never forget— you and those you lead are heroes.

Thom A. Mayer, M.D.
President and
Chief Executive Officer
BestPractices, Inc.
3300 Gallows Road
Falls Church, VA 22042-3300
thom.mayer@inova.com
703/698-2828

Robert J. Cates, M.D.
Chairman
Department of Emergency
Medicine
Inova Fairfax Hospital
3300 Gallows Road
Falls Church, VA 22042-3300
robert.cates@inova.com
703/698-3195

Getting Started:
Why Worry About Customer
Service in Healthcare?

ONE OF THE most intriguing and troubling questions facing healthcare leaders is, *How do I create a meaningful and lasting culture of customer service in my institution?* Improving customer service and patient satisfaction are critical issues in administrative offices and hospital boardrooms across the country. Over twenty books have been written on the application of customer service to healthcare. (Don't they look nice on the bookshelf?) The problem, of course, is that there is plenty of legitimate and genuine concern in the executive suite, but too little practical guidance in the patient care areas where clinical care and customer service are to be provided. The *intention* is almost universally good, but the *execution* is often lacking. Despite posting eloquent mission statements, paying substantial fees to consultants, providing training materials and sophisticated web sites, and delivering appropriately passionate statements at management team meetings to exhort the troops, for many healthcare institutions, when it comes to customer service, the words and the music just don't match.

Why is there such a long shadow between the idea of service excellence and the reality required to bring it to fruition? Why is there such a gap between the proclaimed commitment to and the actual delivery of customer service in healthcare institutions? Noted scholar of organizational behavior Chris Argyris (1993) comments, "For many institutions, the fundamental problem is the dissonance between the espoused strategy and the enacted strategy."

Part of the reason for the dissonance between carefully espoused strategies of customer service and the enacted strategy seen in the patient care areas is that the staff, charged with enacting the strategy and providing the service, can clearly understand why it is important to the CEO, but not why it is important to *them*. As the old story goes,

> The CEO of a large regional healthcare system took one of her key managers to the top of a hill overlooking the city. Pointing down at a ridge just below them, she said, "Imagine a beautiful house sitting atop that ridge, overlooking the city. Can you see it?" "Oh yes, I can see it," said the manager. She continued, "Imagine there is a swimming pool just behind the house, can you see it in your mind?" "Yes, yes I can!" said the manager, getting more excited. "Imagine there is something off to the right of the house—it's a tennis court! Can you see it?" "Yes," said the manager, "I can see it!" The CEO continued, "If this customer service initiative is successful and we continue to increase our market share, someday all of that will be… mine." (Adapted from Belasco and Stayer 1993)

Too often, it is apparent to healthcare providers that customer service initiatives may be great for the leaders and managers of healthcare, but it is often far less apparent why it is good for those who provide that care on a daily basis. We will show you how to make the concept clear.

This book is written for healthcare leaders, but with an understanding that transformation to a culture of service excellence requires not just the *intention* of the leadership but also the constant *attention* of doctors, nurses, radiology technicians, laboratory technicians, registrars, and housekeepers across the organization. For this reason, our intent is to give you direction on how to give them direction to accomplish this. This book, of necessity, presents leaders with an approach to address those who provide service, including numerous clinical examples to use with your staff. While we have found that senior leadership's commitment to service is essential (and we will give you plenty of examples of what you need to do), we have also found that simply exhorting the troops and acting as an example of service are insufficient to create service excellence throughout the organization. The clinicians must be shown *how* this can be done. The bedside examples we give are highly successful strategies to accomplish this. Our greatest hope is that you will finish this book, hand it to your leadership team, and say, "Put this into action!" If you do, you *will* transform your organization.

Many in healthcare feel as if they are "at the ramparts," evoking images of a besieged, embattled industry facing declining revenues, increasing demands, an aging population, healthcare personnel shortages, emergency department crowding and diversion, and the fundamental reality that key providers of service—physicians—are typically neither employed nor controlled by the healthcare system. Into the midst of such difficulties comes the demand for improved customer service and patient satisfaction. Add to this the threat of chemical, biological, nuclear, and explosive terrorism and the rise of new "natural" infectious diseases such as SARS, and healthcare providers may legitimately ask themselves, Is this *really* the time to be focusing on customer service in healthcare?

This honest and straightforward question deserves a frank and direct answer, "Yes!"—but for a reason that is counterintuitive. Having taught the customer service training course (Patient Care Survival Skills) on which this book is based to healthcare providers for 10 years at over 300 healthcare institutions and to over 75,000 healthcare workers, we have found that the most significant challenge to creating a culture of customer service is providing healthcare leaders and the healthcare team a clear and practical understanding of why customer service and patient satisfaction should be important to them. (We know it's important to you—indeed, your job may depend upon it.) To do so, we pose to them—and to you—a simple exercise. Take a moment to think of what your response would be to the following before proceeding further.

The #1 reason to get customer service right in healthcare is _____.

If you are like the thousands of other members of the healthcare team to whom we have given this exercise, your answers generally fall under the following classifications:

- It's better for the patient
- It's better for the family
- It's better for quality care
- It's better for the medical staff
- It's better for market share
- It's better for risk management
- It's better for reimbursement
- It's better for patient safety

All of these are great reasons to get customer service right in healthcare, but who primarily benefits—the service provider or those who lead and manage the organization? As suggested by the first point in the right-hand column, market share improves when customer service improves. Sounds great—but what if I'm a nurse in a busy, overcrowded emergency department. The reward for good customer service is…*more patients*? That doesn't sound like a reward to us.

Any customer service initiative that answers, "Why are we doing this?" with, "Because the boss says so" or "It's good for market share" is doomed to failure. In fact, this is precisely why most customer service initiatives in healthcare either fail or are not sustainable. The fundamental paradox is that, while all of the above responses are certainly true (and excellent reasons for getting customer service right), they still miss the fundamental point:

> *The #1 reason to get customer service right in healthcare is ...*
> ***it makes the job easier.***

It is nearly impossible to effect change in service behaviors in healthcare unless the people providing that care understand this fundamental truth. Anything that is described as customer service should make the job easier. For that reason, there are two simple litmus tests for customer service initiatives and the programs comprising them:

It's called customer service, but...
1. *Does* it make the job easier?
2. *How* does it make the job easier?

If anything that is described as customer service fails either of these two tests, the staff providing the care will fundamentally know that it is not truly customer service. In fact, they understand that things that come labeled as customer service but that do not make their jobs easier are actually *more work*. This is precisely why so many service excellence initiatives in healthcare either fall short of their goals or produce temporary results rather than lasting cultural changes.

How do we communicate this insight in a way that resonates with those who provide care and service to patients on a daily basis? How can we illustrate that customer service makes their job easier? Without a way of creating a widely shared understanding that service excellence works for them—as well as the patient—meaningful and lasting change is unlikely to occur.

We have all seen signs posted at the grocery store or on light poles asking for help in finding lost pets. But you might have missed this one:

> **Lost!**
>
> Small brown dog
> Partially blind
> One leg missing
> Tail has been broken three times and hangs at an
>   unusual angle
> Recently neutered
> Answers to the name "Lucky"

When you introduce customer service programs that do not clearly make your staff's job easier, they don't *feel* "lucky"—they feel *like* "Lucky."

A-TEAM MEMBERS VERSUS B-TEAM MEMBERS

The simplest way to communicate the insight that customer service behaviors actually make the job easier is to pose a single question to your healthcare providers: *Do you offer good customer service?*

Not surprisingly, typical answers include some who enthusiastically answer "Yes!"; some who answer in the affirmative, but less emphatically; and even those whose response is, "No, unfortunately we don't offer consistently good customer service." However, there is also a predictably large group whose answer is neither affirmative nor negative. They believe that the answer to the question is, "It depends." The question of course then becomes, "Upon *what* does it depend?" What are the factors that determine whether we offer good customer service? Again, a simple exercise serves us well in making this determination. Simply pose the following question: *Are there days when you come to work and see the people you are working with and think to yourself, "Bring it on! Whatever we've got to do today, this team of people can make it happen!"*

If they answer with a resounding "Yes!" regardless of whether you work in the OR or the ER, the ICU or medical floor, in house-keeping or the outpatient clinic, this phenomenon is well-known. If you ask them what they call that team, the answer is the same from Maine to Florida and from Alaska to California: the A-team. Question the members of the healthcare team further about the attributes and attitudes of the A-team, and their response is predictable. A-team members are usually described in the following manner:

- Positive
- Proactive
- Confident
- Competent
- Compassionate
- Communicator

- Team player
- Trustworthy
- Teacher
- Does whatever it takes
- Has a sense of humor

This list summarizes the responses from the thousands of health-care providers we've questioned about the attributes of the A-team. Regardless of where they work in the healthcare system, the phenomenon of the A-team is well known but not clearly articulated to those who provide clinical care. This is a team we'd all like to work with—and join. These people make the hard work of providing patient care not only bearable but enjoyable. When you use this exercise, it is important to remember that you don't need to tell them what the A-team attributes are (top down)—they already know and will willingly tell you (bottom up).

However, there is a second part to the above exercise that is equally, if not fundamentally more, important. Ask the staff, *Are there days when you come to work, see who you are working with, and think to yourself, 'Shoot me, shoot me, shoot me!' I can't work with him—I worked with him yesterday! Who in the world makes the schedule around here?!?"*

This team of people—the B-team—is an equally well-known phenomenon among healthcare providers, although they may not have articulated precisely the characteristics that typify the B-team. B-team members can be described by the following terms:

- Negative
- Reactive
- Confused
- Poor communicator
- Lazy
- Late

- Administrator Scrooge
- Constant complainer
- Can't do
- Always surprised
- Nurse Ratched
- Dr. Torquemada

Almost every institution has Nurse Ratcheds (the quintessentially dour and negative nurse of Ken Kesey's *One Flew Over the Cuckoo's Nest*). Many of you are also painfully aware that most institutions also have their Dr. Torquemadas (the Grand Inquisitor of the Spanish Inquisition). Unfortunately, your staff may also think you have an Administrator Scrooge on your management team. An important insight is to recognize that not only do all of you know who Nurse Ratched, Dr. Torquemada, and Administrator Scrooge are in your institutions, but you also know their negative behaviors and faults in infinite detail. In our seminars, we hear about a curious but predictable phenomenon that while staff enjoy articulating the attributes that typify the A-team, they truly *delight* in delineating the B-team behaviors, often shouting them out, laughing as they do so. Regardless of the location where the service is provided, all members of the healthcare team fundamentally understand the phenomenon of the A-team and the B-team in their daily work. They also understand the fundamentally toxic nature of the B-team behaviors, as evidenced by their response to the question, *How many B-team members does it take to destroy an entire shift?* Without exception, every audience shouts the same response— "One!!!"

How can this possibly be? Can one single person destroy the morale of your entire staff in a busy, clinical environment? You bet—

and they do it daily and predictably in your hospitals and healthcare institutions. You know it, and, far more importantly, your staff knows it—they know who these people are, precisely how they act, and the infinite details of their toxic behavior. Any sane person, particularly a leader in healthcare, would ask the only logical question in response to this insight: *Why do we tolerate B-team members and B-team behaviors?*

As one nursing director on a busy clinical unit in an academic medical center told us, "I don't really mind taking care of the patients; they're the reason I went into nursing and management in the first place. It's taking care of the B-team members that wears me out. I don't know how much longer I can do it."

The fundamental problem with the B-team members is not that their behaviors create customer dissatisfaction (although they clearly and predictably do), but that their actions and attitudes are systematically demoralizing the good work provided by the remainder of the healthcare team. If for no other reason, eliminating B-team behaviors is essential to ensuring that employee satisfaction and morale can be maintained at the highest possible level under the admittedly difficult circumstances faced in hospitals and healthcare systems.

Thus, one of the most important insights to take from initiating a customer service program that addresses and eliminates B-team behaviors is not the predictable rise in patient satisfaction scores that will ensue but that A-team members who have tolerated B-team members' behavior for years will understand that leadership and management are *finally* serious about the issue of holding people accountable for their behaviors in a systematic fashion. If you deal with your Nurse Ratched and Dr. Torquemada, your

> A-team behaviors =
> good customer service...
> *And employee satisfaction*
>
> B-team behaviors =
> bad customer service...
> *And employee dissatisfaction*

staff will understand that something is different about *this* customer service program—and that people will be held accountable for service *and* disservice. The problem isn't that the B-team members are harming the patients—they are too smart for that. It's that they are killing morale systematically and daily in the organization. A-team members create and nurture positive morale, even in the face of stress, shortages, and overcrowding. B-team members foment discontent and nurture it in others.

Simply stated, A-team behaviors are good customer service behaviors, not only because they improve patient satisfaction but also because they truly make the job easier on a day-to-day basis. You should hire for these behaviors, train for these behaviors, and reward these behaviors.

B-team behaviors are also predictable and subject to statistical analysis—and predictably produce not only customer dissatisfaction but employee dissatisfaction as well. You all know who Nurse Ratched and Dr. Torquemada are, and you all know their negative behaviors. What remains is to eliminate the B-team behaviors and, regrettably, at times eliminate the B-team members from the ranks. This is not quantum physics or chaos theory—these principles are fundamentally understood by every member of the healthcare team, all of whom recognize the disruptive and negative results of B-team behaviors. The problem is that these behaviors have not been articulated in a clear, concise, and pragmatic way, and leadership and management have not held Nurse Ratched and Dr. Torquemada accountable.

Let's return to the previous question, *Why haven't we gotten rid of the B-team members?* Again, posing a simple question to the staff helps gain fundamental insight into this issue: *Are you an A-team member?*

Everyone to whom this question is posed answers, "Of course, darn right, I am an A-team member and very proud of it!" It is a curious comment on human nature that no one ever says, "I am a B-team member with 20 years of proud provision of miserable service." It just doesn't happen. Why?

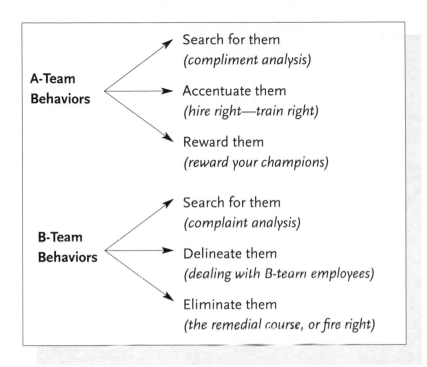

A-Team
Behaviors
- Search for them
  (compliment analysis)
- Accentuate them
  (hire right—train right)
- Reward them
  (reward your champions)

B-Team
Behaviors
- Search for them
  (complaint analysis)
- Delineate them
  (dealing with B-team employees)
- Eliminate them
  (the remedial course, or fire right)

When A-team members look in the mirror, what do they see?
The answer is they see an A-team member, since these people tend to be self-aware, with a clear understanding of what works and what doesn't work, both in the workplace and in their private lives. They know what their A-team behaviors are and how they work, even if that understanding is, to a certain extent, on the subconscious level.

When B-team members look in the mirror, what do they see?
The B-team member sees an A-team member in the reflection, since they do not recognize that their attitudes and behaviors have a poisonous effect on those around them. For B-team members, their behaviors and attitudes work—for them. One of the fundamental roles of leadership and management, in concert with the assistance of the A-team, is to hold the mirror up to the B-team members, letting them see the effect that their behavior has on patients, family, and other members of the healthcare team.

WHY GET CUSTOMER SERVICE RIGHT?

To return to our initial point, the real reason to launch a service excellence initiative is to make the job of healthcare easier. *If it doesn't make the job easier, it isn't really customer service.* The A-team and B-team exercise emphasizes this point clearly. It is important to begin your healthcare customer service journey here, with a fundamental understanding that making the job easier for those who do the job should be the focus of your customer service program—not improving patient satisfaction scores, increasing market share, improving patient safety, or any of the other reasons discussed earlier. As admirable and worthy as these goals are, healthcare is fundamentally a personal service business, delivered daily, even hourly, by those at the bedside. We draw on the critical insight of great psychologists and psychiatrists such as Abraham Maslow, Erik Eriksen, and Victor Frankl, who understood one of the fundamental truths of the human condition: *All meaningful and lasting change is intrinsically motivated.*

A service excellence program that does not show demonstrable and immediate benefit to those charged with delivery of the service will only aggravate the problem. Such top-down programs rarely have more than a transient, fleeting effect. And they often are viewed by staff as a further demand, another stress on a system seemingly stressed to the maximum—simply "more work."

At one of our training sessions, we were speaking to a healthcare system that had previously sent a team to the Disney Institute to create a service excellence program. The nursing director of one of their busiest units said, "Great—Disney comes to healthcare! What's next? The Goofy parking lot? I hope so because I have some suggestions on who can park there!"

The Disney Institute produces excellent customer service. However, unless it can be made clear how such service efforts not only make the job easier but also how they do so, any effort will fail. Those efforts must be translated into healthcare organizations and supported—not simply touted—by leaders in order to truly succeed. That means fostering A-team attitude to drive home the concept of how to get customer service *right*. You do need to hold Nurse Ratched, Dr. Torquemada, and Administrator Scrooge accountable. Admit it—you have been wanting to do that for a very long time. We will show you how to make sure they know they have to "get with the program or get gone."

What Is the Fundamental Problem with the B-Team Members?

Many B-team members seem to be negative, reactive people who begin their day unhappy—and get unhappier by the minute, dragging the morale of patients and staff down with them. Why is this? How can people go to work, day after day, year after year, under such circumstances? Quite simply, *the B-team members are doing a job that isn't their job to do.*

By this we mean that the B-team members have, through multiple pathways and circumstances, ended up doing something for which they are not basically suited; they simply do not have the skills and abilities (largely from an interpersonal standpoint) required to do their job.

I am the father of three boys, and, while the analogies between childrearing and leadership and management can certainly be overdrawn, this story is pertinent to both. Each morning when I drop my sons off at school, they hear the same thing from me: *One more step in the journey of discovering where your deep joy intersects the world's deep needs.* (Understandably, they prefer to take the bus.) Nonetheless, the consistent message is to begin with "your deep joy" as opposed to the "world's deep needs," since all of us must discover what it is we enjoy doing, where it is we enjoy doing it, the kinds of people we enjoy doing it with, and the circumstances under which all of this occurs.

Becoming a doctor or nurse or healthcare executive because "the world needs them" is not a great idea. However, becoming a doctor or a nurse or a healthcare executive because of the fundamental joy in serving people in need is a better match of the "deep joy/deep need" ratio. For many B-team members, they have signed on for a job that is simply not their job to do. They would be better suited either in some other area of healthcare or in an altogether different area of the workforce.

For B-team members, somehow the world is always a surprise to them—they are surprised that there are patients to be taken care of; they are surprised that these patients have needs and expectations that often do not match their own; they are surprised that available resources are taxed to provide such care; they are surprised by... *everything*! One emergency department medical director summed it up nicely:

> I don't understand how these people can be surprised. Many of them have been working in our emergency department for ten years. We see 75,000 visits in a space designed for 40,000 so it is a crazy place. These people have come to work every day for ten years and continue to ask, "Where in the world do all these people come from?" I always tell them, "I need to explain something to you. There is a big red sign above our door that says EMER-GENCY and it has an arrow pointing right at us. I think maybe that's where these people came from."

However, A-team members are rarely surprised, since they have a clear expectation and fundamental knowledge of where their deep joy intersects the world's deep needs. And even when they are surprised, they adapt to it remarkably well, expressing the feelings of one A-team member, "What's my job description? It's to do whatever I have to do to get through the day, to help my patients, to help the people with whom I work. My job description? I guess it's 'Do whatever it takes'."

WHY DO WE CALL THEM "SURVIVAL SKILLS"?

The biggest difference between this book and others on patient satisfaction is its emphasis that *the #1 reason to get customer service right is that it makes the job easier.* As illustrated by the A-team and B-team exercises, healthcare providers can clearly see the practical application of A-team behaviors as fundamental customer service behaviors that not only improve patient and family satisfaction but also improve employee satisfaction in the process.

Why do we call them "Survival Skills"? Because these skills are essential to survive in the complex, complicated, and confusing world of healthcare. Training in these skills—or A-team behaviors—is an investment in the most precious resource in all of healthcare—the providers of healthcare. Herb Kelleher, the colorful and highly successful CEO of Southwest Airlines, was once asked a difficult question: "If you had to choose, would you invest in the employee or in the customer?" His answer came instantly, "In the employee! Because if you take care of the employees, they'll take care of the customers."

The remainder of this book provides practical examples of the A-team behaviors (i.e., Survival Skills), which must be accentuated and rewarded, and B-team behaviors, which must be identified and eliminated.

CUSTOMER SERVICE IS ABOUT YOU

"You" in this case are the healthcare organization providers and administrators. Peter Drucker wisely noted that all service businesses require the voluntary contribution of the provider to choose the type of service that will be created in the interaction with the customer. You cannot force your employees to be nice, professional, friendly, and caring, much less the physicians with whom you work. However, you can show them that all customer service makes their job easier, and all successful customer service initiatives recognize this fundamental truth and put it to work effectively.

How Do You Do It?

How do you create a lasting, meaningful service excellence program? You have to do three simple, yet difficult, things.

1. *There must be a fundamental and universal cultural change.* Whether using the Survival Skills format or any other, the CEO and leadership team must be committed in every action, memo, meeting, speech, and interaction to this transition. The "suits"—the people in the executive suite—must be visible and feel the pain that the frontlines face. As Tom Peters noted 20 years ago, there is tremendous power in the troops seeing you regularly, or MBWA (management by walking around). Round on the patient care units regularly, at least once a week. Put it on your schedule—it's one of the most important things you do. As you walk around, ask your staff this question: *What can I do to make your job easier?* That is the core customer service competency, the #1 reason to get customer service right—to make your (and their) job easier. It takes courage to ask this question, but no service excellence program can succeed without it.

2. *Hire right, and provide universal, practical training to create a service vocabulary visible in daily action.* The hiring of a new employee is the most expensive decision you will ever make as a leader, far more expensive than signing off on a new MRI scanner. The more that employee has frontline contact with patients, the more crucial the hiring decision is (discussed in Chapter 5). Effective, highly practical training must be given to each and every employee. That training must be entertaining,

preferably humorous, and focused on making the employees' jobs easier. Terms like service *recovery*, *A-team vs. B-team*, *empowerment*, *point of impact intervention*, and *scripting* shouldn't reside in policies and procedure manuals—they should reside in the hearts and minds of your leadership team and the doctors, nurses, and other healthcare team members they serve.

3. *Customer service must be a part of the daily experience by rewarding your champions and shooting the stragglers* (and no exceptions for Nurse Ratched and Dr. Torquemada). If service excellence is to be lived in the hallways, elevators, EDs and patient care units, you've got to set the pace by creating meaningful and visible ways of rewarding your champions (see Chapter 6). Simultaneously, you've got to insist that managers hold Dr. Torquemada, Nurse Ratched, and Administrator Scrooge accountable for their B-team behaviors. Otherwise the rest of your staff will understand that there are two sets of rules—one for them and one for Nurse Ratched, Doctor Torquemada, and Administrator Scrooge. Nothing will eviscerate your service excellence faster than the following statements:

    *   "Oh, that's just Nurse Ratched, she's been here forever. We can't do anything about her."
    *   "You just have to learn to tolerate Dr. Torquemada. He's the hospital's biggest admitter."
    *   "Administrator Scrooge was here when they laid the first stone. He always talks about customer service, but he *never* comes out to the patient care areas. Learn to deal with him."

As illustrated in the B-team exercise, your staff knows in infinite detail who these people are and how they behave. They are waiting for someone with the courage to hold the B-team members accountable. It needs to be you. It needs to be *now*.

SURVIVAL SKILLS SUMMARY

While CEO and senior management commitment to customer service is essential, your staff has to understand the following:

- The #1 reason to get customer service right is it makes the job easier!
- The customer service litmus test is if it doesn't make the job easier for your staff, it isn't *really* customer service.
- The A-team is a group of people who are admired and respected because their behaviors and attributes make life easier not just for the patient but also for those with whom they work.
- Discover who the A-team members are in your organization and learn what they are doing.
- Use the A-team/B-team exercise to demonstrate to your staff that A-team behaviors are simply good customer service that will make their jobs easier.
- The B-team members' attitudes and attributes not only make life miserable for the patient but also for your staff. Discovering who the B-team members are is, strangely, much easier than identifying the A-team members.
- How many B-team members does it take to destroy an entire shift? One!
- Identify A-team members and the skills they use—accentuate them, insist on them, and reward them.
- Identify B-team members and behaviors—then eliminate either the behaviors or the people.
- Identify your Nurse Ratched, Dr. Torquemada, and Administrator Scrooge—let them know it's time to get with the program or get gone.
- Creating customer service is as easy as 1-2-3:
  1. Make it clear that a fundamental and universal cultural change toward service excellence is happening.

2. Hire right, train right, and create a service vocabulary for your staff.
3. Make it a part of the daily experience—and shoot the stragglers!

REFERENCES

Argyris, C. 1993. *Knowledge for Action: A Guide to Overcoming Barriers to Organizational Change*. San Francisco: Jossey-Bass.

Belasco, J. A., and R. C. Stayer. 1993. *The Flight of the Buffalo*. New York: Warner Books.

MORE ON THIS

Berry, L. L. 1999. *Discovering the Soul of Service: The Nine Drivers of Sustainable Business Success*. New York: The Free Press.
Len Berry is the preeminent source concerning the science of service. This study of 14 service industry leaders has many lessons for healthcare.

Block, P. 2002. *The Right Use of Power: How Stewardship Replaces Leadership*. Louisville, CO: Sounds True.
Audio/CD available at PeterBlock.com.

Patterson, K., J. Grenny, R. McMillan, A. Switzler, and S. Covey. 2002. *Crucial Conversations: Tools for Talking When the Stakes Are High*. New York: McGraw-Hill.

Peters, T. 2003. *Re-imagine!* New York: Dorling Kindersly.
The latest from the incomparable Tom Peters—a great resource and a great read.

CHAPTER 2

Are They Patients,
or Are They Customers?

AS ACCOUNTABILITY FOR patient satisfaction becomes more prevalent, and as healthcare providers increasingly hold themselves more accountable for such skills, one of the most difficult dilemmas is developing a concise and meaningful answer to the question you all face regarding the people in your care: *Are they patients or are they customers?*

The majority of physicians, nurses, and healthcare workers that we have encountered in our research indicate that the answer to this question is straightforward—individuals seeking care are patients, not customers. Common reactions include:

- "This is not Nordstrom or Wal-Mart—they are patients, not customers."
- "Stop calling them patients? Start calling them customers? Give me a break! Better yet, give me some nausea medicine!"

Your clinical staff clearly sees those they care for as patients. But are they customers as well? "Customers" could refer to a diverse range of participants in the healthcare process, including patients, family members, payers, employers, and even the providers of healthcare themselves, who are internal customers to the process. However, for the purposes of our discussion, let's restrict the use of the term to those who are the direct recipients of the healthcare provided.

So... what are they? To stimulate discussion of this question, we use an exercise that helps healthcare professionals realize that they have their own inherent and intuitive definitions of customers and patients, even if those definitions have not yet been clearly articulated. We ask them to imagine a gauge with a needle that will point toward either "patient" or "customer," depending solely on their reactions to specific clinical scenarios.

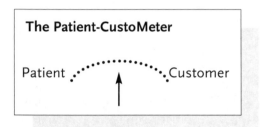

The following are three clinical scenarios, in this case drawn from the emergency department (ED). After reading each scenario, we pose the simple question, "Is this a patient or a customer?"

Scenario 1. A 65-year old woman presents to the ED with severe, intermittent chest pain that began one hour ago. The patient rates her pain as a 9 on a scale of 10, which is unrelieved by the nitroglycerine given by the paramedics en route. Her EKG clearly shows an acute anterior myocardial infarction. *Is this a patient or a customer?*

Scenario 2. A three-year old child presents to the ED at 3 o'clock in the morning, having been seen by her pediatrician at 3 o'clock in the afternoon, where a diagnosis of an ear infection was made and the patient was started on antibiotics and given fever control instructions. Now the patient has a temperature of 99.2°F (normal being 98.6°F), and the parents say they "can't get the fever down," despite the fact that no fever medication has been given and the antibiotic prescription hasn't been filled. *Is this a patient or a customer?*

Scenario 3. This scenario is precisely the same as Scenario 2 with one exception—this child is your own. *Is this a patient or a customer?*

Despite asking these questions of thousands of healthcare professionals from diverse backgrounds living in numerous geographic locations, the results are absolutely consistent. The woman in scenario 1 is universally described as a patient, whereas the child in scenario 2 is described as a customer (with the parents being identified as the primary customer). Scenario 3 invariably causes healthcare professionals to question whether they would classify their own child as a patient or a customer. As we hear from many respondents, "The needle waivers a little on that third scenario." When asked why they rate the woman as a patient and the child (and his parents) as customers, the results are also highly predictable, as described below:

Patient
- Acutely ill or injured
- Dependent on physician
- Power/control with clinician
- Less choice
- Technical expertise required
- Higher satisfaction for clinician
- High clarity of treatment required
- Time dependent

Customer
- Less severely ill
- Independent
- Power/control with customer
- More choice
- Service skills required
- Lower satisfaction for clinician
- Less clarity of treatment required
- Service dependent

Patients are more acutely ill, feel quite sick, have little or no choice in where they seek their healthcare, and are largely dependent on the healthcare practitioner to deliver technical expertise in a time-dependent fashion. In "patient" relationships the healthcare professional is the primary locus of power and has control during the (fundamentally) clinical encounter.

Customers are less acutely ill or injured, have substantial choice in where their healthcare is provided, are more independent, and have substantially more power and control over the healthcare encounter than do patients. The needs of customers are more service dependent, while those of the patient are more clinically dependent.

It is important to note that healthcare professionals tell us without exception that they feel a high degree of clarity in knowing how to take care of patients, who primarily require technical expertise to care for their illnesses or injuries. However, most healthcare professionals are far less clear about how to approach the customer, largely because of the lack of specific and detailed training in addressing such needs and expectations. This exercise helps your staff recognize that they subconsciously and tacitly ask the question, "Is this a patient or a customer?" every time they pick up a patient's chart. They make that determination by using a simple, straightforward, but unwritten diagnostic rule known intuitively to everyone in healthcare:

Are They Patients, or Are They Customers?

The more horizontal they are, the more they're patients.
The more vertical they are, the more they're customers.

This diagnostic rule has virtually 100 percent sensitivity and specificity—in other words, it will never fail you. Those who are horizontal (or nearly so) are dependent on the delivery of technical skills, often in an expert and rapid fashion. Those who are more vertical have more control in the provider-patient/customer relationship and are often unafraid to exercise that control, sometimes to the consternation of the healthcare provider.

HIGH VERSUS LOW EXPECTATIONS

Our research indicates that the role of expectations is a crucial one in healthcare. To illustrate that role, we ask course participants who has higher expectations—the lady with the heart attack or the parents of the child with a fever. The answer is always "the parents." What are the parents' (customers') expectations? They want reassurance that their child is not acutely ill so that they can go home, put the child to bed, and get back to sleep. What is it that the lady (patient) wants? Well, she wants to live.

Let's make sure that we have this right: the parents want fever control instructions and reassurance so they can sleep—and staff consider that "high expectations." The lady is dying and the providers are going to ensure that she continues to live—and consider that "low expectations." Intuitively, this seems odd. However, without exception, these are the responses from every healthcare institution across the country. How can someone who is dying have low expectations? How can giving reassurance to parents be a high expectation? Is this fundamentally flawed reasoning?

No, because what that lady is "buying"—life-saving care— providers love to "sell" and are *highly trained* in the delivery thereof. Providers enjoy taking care of patients who are that severely ill, precisely because it is a skill in which they have a high degree of confidence. Saving lives—that's what they signed up for! Ask your ED or critical care staff, "What if the lady gets *really* sick? What if she has a cardiac arrest?" Their answer? "Cool!"

Let's be clear here—they don't *want* her to arrest (it's not like they're going to stand on her oxygen hose or anything like that). It's that they love to take care of the critically ill, they're *very* good at it, and it is personally and professionally satisfying.

The parents' expectations —reassurance that the child is okay— is not part of the curriculum for our medical schools or nursing schools, and our healthcare institutions generally don't address it well in orientation or in-services. The parents' expectations are "high" because they are expectations providers have not been trained to meet in an explicit fashion. Further, they seem like high expectations because not nearly as much satisfaction is derived from giving fever control instructions as from saving lives. That shouldn't be surprising—that's human nature.

So which is it, are they patients or are they customers? Is it the art or the science? Is it the name ("Mrs. Gazungas in room 4") or the disease ("The belly pain in room 5")? At one academic medical center with an international reputation, we overheard a female resident say to one of her colleagues, "I just saw your appendix." Now, either she had flunked anatomy or she had seen a *patient* with suspected appendicitis. *All language has meaning.* Therefore, language in your institution should reflect the commitment to the patient, not the disease.

Is the job to care or to cure? Is it the journey or is it the destination? We travel the country speaking about customer service. How much credit do you think we give the airlines for getting us from point A to point B and not killing us? How about *none*—we expect that. Your patients expect excellent clinical care (the destination). But they also expect excellent service (the journey). The destination is assumed—the journey is usually how service is judged. Is it the vertical or the horizontal? Is it the ER or the PR? The answer, of course, is that it is always, to varying degrees, both.

Customers ————————▶	Patients
80% to 90%	10% to 20%
These people are the *price* you pay...	for the *privilege* of taking care of these people.

Take the "Are they patients or are they customers?" exercise further. Say to your healthcare providers and leaders, "You told us who were patients and who were customers. During a typical day at your job, how many patients do you see and how many customers?" Even in a busy emergency department or trauma/critical care unit, it is not uncommon to hear ratios of 80 to 90 percent customers and 10 to 20 percent patients. If that is your staff's perception (and it clearly is), then the following is also true:

Most providers go into healthcare to make a difference in people's lives—that is their "deep joy, deep need." The sicker the patient is (within the definition and confines of the specific healthcare areas), the better the providers like them. (What nurse is really enthused about a fully ambulatory "customer" who hits the call light every 17 seconds?) A tremendous amount of job and personal satisfaction comes from caring for those who are severely ill and injured and somewhat less from those with high, unreasonable expectations.

GOOD PATIENTS?

After the "Are they patients or are they customers?" exercise, we also ask the staff to help us define what, in their minds, constitutes a "good patient." It might surprise—or shock—you to learn that the responses we get as we travel around the country are summarized as follows:

- In restraints
- Gagged
- Handcuffed
- Orphan (no family)
- Compliant (wants it "our" way)

- Speaks "our" language
- Doesn't come back
- In and out fast
- Wants only one thing

The single adjective that is always listed by every audience is "compliant." Ask them what that means and they'll tell you, "It means that they do what they're told, they follow directions." The great psychologist Abraham Maslow suggested that the base of the hierarchy of needs includes issues of power and control as fundamental needs for human beings. If this exercise is any indicator, healthcare providers enjoy situations in which they have power and control over patients. When people are horizontal—patients—the power and control reside with the healthcare provider and those who manage those providers. As the patient becomes more vertical, they become more of a customer, and the power/control curve slides toward them (the customer). The entire list of good patients (while humorous—if not shocking—to read) gives credence to Maslow's insight, but the exercise lends itself to a deeper understanding.

YOUR ENTREPRENEURIAL VENTURE

If your staff's response to the question, "What makes a good patient?" is similar to the one above (and it will be), it is important to make an additional point to healthcare leaders and providers:

What if this was not healthcare, but your own business, your own entrepreneurial venture? How would you define "good?"

To make this point, ask your staff to consider the following scenario. Imagine that we were going to give each of you your own entrepreneurial venture and that your entire future, your retirement, your benefits, your salary, your savings plan, and your ability to send your kids to college are dependent on that entrepreneurial venture. The entrepreneurial venture is a chicken franchise—Bucket O' Clucks. What are the factors that would guide the success of your chicken franchise? Compare your customer requirements to what you told us constituted good patients.

"In restraints, gagged, and handcuffed" wouldn't make any sense at all (unless your chicken franchise was serving incarcerates). If you have a chicken franchise, you don't want orphans because you want them to bring the entire family (that's why signs at restaurants say "Buses welcome!"). How about "Speaks 'our' language"? In your chicken franchise you don't care what language they speak—they can point to the chicken. "Doesn't come back"? If it were your entrepreneurial venture you would want them to come back for breakfast, lunch, and dinner. "In and out fast"? No, you would want them to linger and come back for seconds. "Wants only one thing"? Of course not, how about some side dishes with that chicken? And a nice slice of pie or cheesecake? Finally, "Compliant—wants it our way"? As Burger King says, "Have it *your* way." The point is simple—if this were your entrepreneurial venture, if your livelihoods completely depended on it, in many ways you would want the opposite of what, with gallows humor, your staff might list as good patients.

Take the exercise one step further and ask your staff how many years they have worked at your healthcare institution. Five years? Ten years? Fifteen years? Twenty years? Some have worked at your hospital for as long as twenty-five years. It might surprise you how many hands go up for over ten years. The punchline? "I have news for those of you who have worked here over ten years—this *is* your chicken franchise." They will never miss the point that this is a business that they fundamentally need to grow and treat as if it were their own entrepreneurial venture. Their futures *do* depend on the success of this enterprise. While they may not *own* it (in the entrepreneurial sense), they "own it" in the sense that their futures, hopes, and deep joy are invested in its success.

WHAT PERCENT PATIENT AND WHAT PERCENT CUSTOMER?

Practical experience and common sense tell you what textbooks do not:

> *If someone is about 80 percent patient (horizontal),*
> *he or she is also about 20 percent customer (vertical).*

The relationship could be described graphically with the "customer percentage" on the vertical axis and the "patient percentage" on the horizontal. It would look something like this:

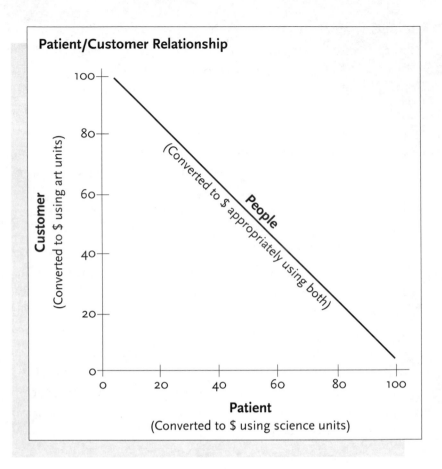

Patient/Customer Relationship

Customer (Converted to $ using art units) — vertical axis: 0, 20, 40, 60, 80, 100

Patient (Converted to $ using science units) — horizontal axis: 0, 20, 40, 60, 80, 100

(Converted to $ appropriately using both)

People

It's a fairly simple, but straightforward, concept: Adding the % patient and % customer = 100%. The corollary to this is: *Wouldn't it work well if we treated the "% patient" with technical skills and the "% customer" with customer service skills?*

For example, let's say we estimate that the child from scenario 2 (the three-year-old at 3 a.m.) is about 80 percent customer and about 20 percent patient. That implies we should treat the 80 percent customer with service skills (A-team behaviors). It might sound like this:

Triage nurse: "I have kids of my own and I know how hard it can be when your child is ill. However, the good news is that his temperature is actually normal, so he doesn't have what we define medically as a fever, even though his head may feel hot to the touch. Let's have the doctor examine him, but it's very likely you'll be able to go home and get some rest once he's been evaluated and treated."

Combining the 80 percent customer with the 20 percent patient might sound like this:

> *Emergency physician*: "I've examined your child very thoroughly and I agree with your pediatrician that he has an ear infection, but I see no evidence of a more serious illness, such as meningitis. We should continue the antibiotic and the fluids and medications you've been giving to control his temperature. You've done a great job, since his temperature is normal. We'll give him another dose of antibiotic to boost his blood level. Go home, get some rest, and I'd suggest calling your doctor in the morning. Do you have any questions about any of this?"

The problem with American healthcare is that we have been terrific at treating the patient/technical side and fairly miserable in treating the customer/service side. One of the main focuses we present in our Survival Skills seminars is the necessity to understand the following: *Just as every patient has a clinical diagnosis, they have a customer service diagnosis as well.*

This leads us to the first Survival Skill: *Make the Customer Service Diagnosis (as well as the clinical diagnosis) and Offer the Right Treatment.*

Nearly a century ago, Sir William Osler made the same point in a different way: *It is more important to know what sort of patient has the disease than what sort of disease the patient has.*

The patient-customer equation, while extremely helpful in understanding the customer service diagnosis, is not a static equation. Your staff can't just make both the customer service diagnosis as well as the clinical diagnosis, treat both, and declare victory. As the patient (and their loved ones) journey through the healthcare system, it is the fundamental goal to move them from the horizontal to the vertical. As that journey progresses, their needs fundamentally change from those of a patient to those of a customer. When a patient presents to the emergency department in cardiac arrest, she is nearly 100 percent horizontal. As the providers resuscitate her and transfer her to the cardiac care unit, the "axis rotates" as she becomes more vertical. When it's time for discharge from the hospital, the patient has happily completed the journey to being nearly 100 percent vertical. Providers need to continue to ask themselves, *Has the patient-customer axis rotated today?*

Finally, always remember to ask (and answer) the following:

- Are they patients or are they customers? *They are always both, to varying degrees.*
- Do we need clinical skills or customer service skills? *We always need both, depending on the customer service diagnosis and the clinical diagnosis.*

Making the customer service (as well as the clinical) diagnosis and offering the right treatment is the subject of the next chapter, as we move from the "why?" of healthcare customer service to the details of "how?"

SURVIVAL SKILLS SUMMARY

- In every clinical encounter in your healthcare system, your staff subconsciously asks themselves, "Is this a patient or a customer?"
- The more horizontal they are (acutely ill, dependent, less choice, less vocal), the more they are a *patient*. The more vertical they are (less acutely ill, independent, more choice, more vocal), the more they are a *customer*.
- As the patient's health improves, he or she becomes more of a customer. Thus, the axis rotates from horizontal to vertical.

- Use the "Are they a patient or are they a customer?" exercise to help your staff understand this important issue.
- Help your staff understand the need to ask, "Has this person's patient/customer axis rotated today?"
- Almost perversely, staff think that patients (people who are very sick) have "low expectations," while customers (people who are more well) have "high expectations." They feel this way because they are well trained and skilled at meeting patient expectations, or they feel they are poorly trained and don't enjoy meeting customer expectations. This is why service excellence requires skills training.
- Are they patients or are they customers? *They are always both—to varying degrees in the course of their journey* through our healthcare system.
  The % patient added to the % customer always equals 100%.
- Treat the "% patient" with technical skills and the "% customer" with service excellence skills.

MORE ON THIS

These short articles from both the medical and business literature range from defining patients and customers to strategies for change in healthcare.

Berwick, D. M. 2003. "Disseminating Innovations in Healthcare." *Journal of the American Medical Association* 289 (15): 1969–75.

Mayer, T., and R. J. Cates. 1999. "Service Excellence in Health Care." *Journal of the American Medical Association* 282 (13): 1281–83.

Mayer, T., R. Cates, M. J. Mastorovich, and D. L. Royalty. 1998. "Emergency Department Patient Satisfaction: Customer Service Training Improves Patient Satisfaction and Ratings of Physician and Nurse Skill." *Journal of Healthcare Management* 43 (5): 427–40.

CHAPTER 3

The First Survival Skill:
Making the Customer Service Diagnosis
(in Addition to the Clinical Diagnosis)
and Offering the Right Treatment

AT THIS POINT, we move from the "why?" of healthcare customer service to the "how?" of implementation. In the previous chapter, we showed that every patient has both a clinical diagnosis (requiring technical expertise) and a customer service diagnosis (requiring service excellence skills). In healthcare, we need to diagnose—and treat—both. Until now, we have been training for technical excellence but only measuring customer satisfaction.

Consider the following scenario of "Where do I hit with the hammer?"

A man had a car that looked great but made an awful noise when he drove it. This car made so much noise that people would point to it as it drove by and put their fingers in their ears. The guy took it to a garage and asked the mechanic if he could fix it. The mechanic looked at it, listened to it, and said, "I think I can help you."

The mechanic put the car on the rack with the engine running, raised it in the air, and peered up underneath for a minute or two.

He reached over to his tool box, pulled out a ten-pound ballpeen hammer, and swung it in a broad arc, hitting the car as hard as he possibly could. Suddenly, the engine purred and the car was fixed! The mechanic brought the car down, drove it around the block, and it stayed fixed. He wrote out a bill and handed it to the customer. The bill was for $75. The customer cried, "You charged me $75 to hit my car with a ballpeen hammer?!?"

"No," the mechanic said. "I charged you 5 bucks for hitting your car with a hammer. I charged you 70 bucks for knowing *where* to hit it with the hammer."

The first Survival Skill recognizes that we need to hit not just on the technical aspect of offering the right clinical treatment but also on the customer service aspect as well.

WHERE ARE WE?

One of the first efforts in a service excellence initiative is to develop a clear sense of where you are when you start. After all, how can you know where you're going unless you know where you are? In 1994, we began our customer service excellence journey in just that fashion, by asking patients what they thought of the customer service in our emergency department. We used questionnaires, focus groups, complaint analysis, telephone surveys—anything to discover what the community thought of our customer service skills at that time. We wanted to know, *Where are we?*

What we heard from patients/customers is that technical excellence is widely known—but expected. In other words, if you ask your staff about patients who have complaints, staff will likely respond, "But I made the right diagnosis and I gave them the right treatment." And they will be correct; however, while patient safety is clearly an extremely important issue in healthcare, making the right diagnosis and offering the right treatment *alone* will not suffice when it comes to how carefully and deeply patients and their families assess your services.

When providers tell you they have made the right diagnosis and the right treatment, you may want to say, "Do you think they would come to our hospital if they thought they were going to get the *wrong* diagnosis and treatment? They can go to our competitor hospitals if they want that!" The fact is that technical excellence (and the stress is on excellence, not just competence in today's competitive healthcare environment), is a *necessary condition* for healthcare success—it must be there for success to occur. However, it is not a *sufficient condition*—it is not enough to ensure that success occurs. Your patients will probably tell you what our patients told us in the second part of the "Where are we?" dialog: Although technical excellence is widely known (but expected), *caring* competence is not as high.

If you tell your staff that their caring competence is not as high as their technical competence, have you just told them that they don't care about their patients? No, of course not. However, it often *feels* to them as if you have. The point is simple—ask yourself how much training your staff had in medical school, residency, nursing school, hospital orientation, and in-service education in technical skills and making the clinical diagnosis and the correct treatment. Now, ask how much training they get in caring competence—the customer service skills necessary and largely expected by all of your patients/customers. If your institution is like most, over 90 percent of the training and ongoing education are geared toward technical aspects; although certainly extremely important, too often such education is to the exclusion of training in service skills. The bottom line is that you are going to be judged by both, so you must train for both, in a systematic and rigorous fashion.

MAKING THE CUSTOMER SERVICE DIAGNOSIS

The first Survival Skill involves making the customer service diagnosis *in addition* to the clinical diagnosis—not to the *exclusion* of the clinical diagnosis. Every patient needs to be both effectively diagnosed and treated if healthcare service success is to occur. Your staff is actually very good at figuring out what the customer service diagnosis is—they simply haven't discussed it in an upfront fashion. To illustrate, do this simple exercise below with your staff. Tell them that you will show them, in the left-hand column, a common clinical diagnosis or chief complaint, and simply ask them what the biggest fear or concern—the customer service diagnosis—the patient or family has concerning this clinical diagnosis or chief complaint.

Clinical Diagnosis	Fear—Customer Service Diagnosis
Pediatric fever	"Does my child have meningitis?"
Chest pain	"Have I had a heart attack?"
Abdominal pain	"Do I have appendicitis?"
	"Do I have cancer?" (if the patient is over 50 years of age)
Facial laceration	"Will I have a scar?"
	"Am I going to get a shot?"
	"Will it get infected?"

As you can see from these examples, making both the clinical diagnosis and the customer service diagnosis are subject to reasonable expectations and diagnosis by your staff. The problem is not their ability to figure out what the customer service diagnosis is; it is that they have never been trained to do so, much less how to treat these diagnoses. Encourage your leadership team to use these examples and others that they may develop to help understand more clearly not just what the technical clinical diagnosis is but what the customer service concerns are as well. Look carefully in your institution to see if both the customer service diagnosis and the clinical diagnosis are being made—and met!

ANTICIPATING EXPERIENCES FROM THE CUSTOMER'S VIEWPOINT

As you and your leadership team make your rounds, try to view healthcare not from the perspective of the one providing it but from the perspective of the one receiving it. Many of our processes and systems in healthcare clearly have not been designed from the customer's viewpoint, but instead from the viewpoint of those providing that care. Patient-focused care, the Plaintree model, indeed the majority of service excellence initiatives, all understand the need to design systems and processes from the patient/customer viewpoint, rather than from the provider's. Further, make sure your staff understands that most patients and their families are confused, concerned, and sometimes in pain when they cross your threshold. You should expect that and anticipate their needs in advance; this will make it much easier to meet those needs.

Creating Power and Control Options

As discussed earlier, the psychologist Abraham Maslow devised his hierarchy of needs with a clear understanding that the base of that hierarchy involves fundamental issues of power and control (physiologic and psychologic safety needs) in our daily lives. What does this have to do with the concept of *Is this a patient or is this a customer?* Ask your staff this simple question:

> *In an encounter that is nearly 100 percent patient,*
> *who primarily has the power and control?*
> *The patient? Or those providing care to the patient?*

Your staff will understand that when someone is nearly 100 percent horizontal, the power and control lie with those who are providing the care. The more desperately ill or injured a patient is, the more he or she is perfectly willing to give power and control to those to whom their healthcare is entrusted. But what about the corollary:

In an encounter that is nearly 100 percent customer,
who has the power and control? The customer?
Or those who provide healthcare to the customer?

When someone is nearly 100 percent vertical, they primarily have the power and control. Do your staff like that? The answer is "No!" Why? Because your staff are bad people? No—it is because they are people, and all people dislike situations in which they lack power and control, as Maslow (1998) so correctly pointed out.

To effectively make the customer service diagnosis and offer the right treatment, everyone in healthcare must understand this dynamic of power and control. The more horizontal someone is, the more he or she is willing to *give up* power and control; the more vertical, the more he or she *insists on* power and control. Patients are actually fighting for the vertical, trying not just to get better but to regain power and control over their lives. Staff must understand this and work with the patient as the horizontal-to-vertical axis shifts during the course of the patient's journey through the healthcare system. As patients become more vertical, they must be given increasing degrees of power and control. Giving the patient power and control options works, for you and for them. Examples abound in healthcare, all with evidence of better satisfaction and better outcomes for the patient. These include:

• Better results when prostate cancer patients help choose whether surgery or radiation is their best treatment.
• Better compliance with taking medication (with fewer side effects) when patients are given a "voice in the choice" of medication among several with similar efficiency.
• Better compliance and earlier resolution of symptoms when patients or parents have a choice of antibiotic therapy.

- Better nutrition when patients are given the opportunity to select from a broader list of dietary options (or even the time they eat).

Clearly, one of the most significant sources of power in health-care is information. Good information is good customer service!

EXPECTATION CREATION

Let your patients know what to expect. The more they know what to expect, the more they feel in (some) control—and the happier they are. Give them previews. You've seen previews in the movie theater—use that concept with your patients to give them a taste of what's to come.

Expectation creation lets the patient/customer know what to expect within reasonably specified time frames. The Walt Disney Corporation is a past master of the art and science of expectation creation. Think about the last time you were at a Disney theme park. Remember the sign that said *Wait from here is 40 minutes?*

When you see the sign, you have a couple of options. First, you can decide 40 minutes is too long and move on to the next attraction, perhaps returning later when the line may be shorter. Or you can jump into line and check your watch so you know how close you are to the head of the line. Disney then sets about turning you this way and that as you proceed through the line. Often video monitors preview the ride or change scenery to make the time pass more quickly—all designed to keep you informed, mark your progress, and make the wait easier. The folks at Disney know that *it's not how much time you spend, it's how you spend the time.*

Finally it's your turn and you're on the ride. You glance at your watch and realize, "It's only been 34 minutes. Great!" You might even think, "We got in faster than 40 minutes—we must have gotten the VIP treatment!"

The Disney experts in expectation creation told us they actually *expect* that 92 percent of people will be on the ride within 32 minutes of the time they pass the sign. They create an expectation they expect not only to meet but to exceed. What does this have to do with healthcare? Next time you are on administrative rounds, ask one of the inpatients, "What's going to happen to you today? What's on the agenda? Where are you in your journey back to health?" The vast majority of the patients in your hospital have no clue—not because they are less than intelligent and curious, but because you are not using *expectation creation* to let them know where they are and what to expect.

What about exceeding expectations? How do you do that? Like Disney, your staff can reasonably estimate how long a process should normally take, then give the patient an expanded estimate. For example, if your staff believes that a chest x-ray will take about 45 minutes to complete under normal conditions, they should tell the patient, "I believe the chest x-ray will take an hour to an hour and 15 minutes. But I'll see if I can move it along faster for you." When the chest film is done in 45 minutes (or even 55 minutes) the patient is happy. Expectation creation has given the patient a sense of power and control—by using information. Expectation creation is a skill at which everyone in healthcare needs to be adept.

VERBAL SKILLS AND COMPLAINT/COMPLIMENT ANALYSIS

Many of the best examples of making the customer service diagnosis and offering the right treatment involve a combination of verbal skills and simple courtesies. Examples include:

Situation	Verbal Skill
Patient/family look lost in hallway	"May I help you find where you're going? It can be a bit confusing around here."

Elevator etiquette	"After you, please." No discussions of patient care or sensitive information on elevators. "Let me move over to make room for you."
Child with laceration in ED triage	"You've come to the right place; we take care of these all the time."
Patient checking in for elective procedure	"Welcome, Mr. Smith, we've been expecting you."
All patients	"Thank you for choosing our hospital and trusting us with your care."

As your customer service initiative grows and gains speed and momentum, your staff will develop and recognize more and more of these verbal skills, which are nothing more (or less) than A-team behaviors, all of which work by making your job easier—no matter who "you" are. These verbal A-team behaviors should be discussed at every staff meeting to engender group— not individual—learning. This is also why all complaints and compliments must be discussed and analyzed at staff meetings.

Patient Compliment ⟶	What were the A-team behaviors that generated the compliment? ⟶	Celebrate, accentuate, and circulate them.
Patient Complaint ⟶	What were the B-team behaviors that generated the complaint? ⟶	Identify, isolate, and eliminate them.

Although complaint and compliment analysis (with trending over time) and instant feedback to the staff are essential, it is probably the most neglected concept in service excellence. As we discuss in the next chapter, service recovery is crucial. Not only do we hear the voice of the customer but we also have a chance to give that feedback instantly to our staff.

SURVIVAL SKILLS SUMMARY

• Patients and their family are widely aware of our technical excellence—but this excellence is *expected*.
• Our caring competence—our customer service skills—are generally not as highly rated as our technical skills. Orientation to most healthcare in this country is much more heavily geared toward technical skills, with much less emphasis on service skills. Without neglecting the former, find a way to place considerably more emphasis on training for customer service, both in orientation and in ongoing education.
• Just as every patient has a technical, clinical diagnosis, they also have a customer service diagnosis.
• The first Survival Skill is making the customer service diagnosis and offering the right treatment.
• Anticipate experiences from the customer's viewpoint and change your systems to reflect this customer focus.
• Help your staff learn to create power and control options for both patients and customers.
• Expectation creation is a powerful tool—put it to work.
• Use compliment analysis (A-team behaviors) and complaint analysis (B-team behaviors) to identify verbal skills that produce service excellence.
• Develop and use scripts to accentuate A-team behaviors.

REFERENCE

Maslow, A. H. 1998. *Maslow on Management*. New York: Wiley.

MORE ON THIS

Berry, L. L., and N. Bendapudi. 2003. "Clueing in Customers." *Harvard Business Review* 81 (2): 100–106.
Service from the customer's perspective at the Mayo Clinic, as seen through the eyes of a legend in service writings.

CHAPTER 4

The Second Survival Skill: Negotiating Agreement and Resolution of Expectations

AS A HEALTHCARE leader, how often do you negotiate? Every day, twice a day, four times a day, all day? It depends, of course, but few would argue that negotiation is a key core competency for leaders and managers, as well as for bedside providers of healthcare. Of course you negotiate contracts, payment rates, issues between departments, and other areas of a legal nature, but we are referring to something more fundamental and far more frequent in healthcare. Throughout your healthcare system, negotiations regarding patient care are occurring daily, hourly, even by the minute. Think about the following; don't they all involve negotiation as a core competency?

- *Charge nurse to staff nurses*: "I need someone to take this patient."
- *Shift supervisor to the registration bed board*: "The emergency department needs three critical care beds ASAP."
- *Operating suite supervisor to CEO*: "Dr. Smith wants more block OR time or he says he'll take his business elsewhere."

- *Chief of medicine to director of radiology*: "Why can't we get the radiology reports on the chart (or the computer) before 8 a.m. when the doctors round on their patients?"
- *CEO to department director*: "Our institution has committed to service excellence throughout the organization. I've noticed that your unit's customer service scores have been trending downward. I've asked my assistant to block a couple of hours so we can discuss this in some depth. For part of that time, I've asked Jane Smith to join us, since her unit has had great scores, so she can share some ideas that could be of help."
- *Emergency physician to a patient's family*: "I know you feel your mother needs to be admitted to the hospital, but her illness is not one that usually meets the criteria that we think of for admission. Why don't I discuss it with her physician so he can make a final decision?"

All of these scenarios involve negotiations among members of the healthcare team. Moreover, there is an even more common negotiation that occurs thousands of times a day in every healthcare system in this country, whether in the emergency department, the inpatient units, outpatient settings, or even long-term care: The negotiation between patients/customers and caregivers about their expectations for healthcare.

The patient has one set of expectations while those in healthcare often have another, somewhat different, set of expectations. Without training in negotiation skills, how can we hope to resolve these differences and expectations? This chapter addresses the second Survival Skill: *Negotiating Agreement and Resolution of Expectations*. However, an in-depth treatment of the rich and fascinating study of negotiations requires more space than this brief chapter allows. For that, we refer you to the "More on This" section at the end of the chapter for some excellent resources on negotiation.

In our view, the finest book on negotiation is the simple yet nuanced text by Fisher, Ury, and Patton, *Getting to Yes*. (Based on their experience with the Harvard Negotiation Project, the book is brimming with insight and delineates the quintessential approach to successful negotiation.) Perhaps the most important aspect of negotiation as listed by Fisher, Ury, and Patton is one of the four central points of *Getting to Yes*—the concept of inventing options for mutual gain. Many people define negotiation as "win-win" or "meeting in the middle"—or, more simply, "compromise." While these definitions sound great, how do they work in action? Consider the following interchange.

> *Nursing supervisor*: "I need you to take this patient—the emergency department is getting slammed!"
> *Med-surg charge nurse*: "We can't, we just took two patients four hours ago."
> *Charge nurse*: "Okay … how about taking half of a patient?"

In this situation, meeting in the middle, meeting halfway, or compromising doesn't seem to work. What we need to do is to *invent options for mutual gain*—particularly the patient's gain. Consider the following negotiation around the same issue. The parentheses are used to emphasize the power of carefully selected negotiation language and obviously would not be a part of what was actually said.

> *Nursing supervisor to med-surge nurse*: "Julie (using people's names is powerful), I need your help with a critical issue we have" (enlisting help versus giving orders, defining the importance, and using the plural pronoun). The ED is getting slammed (simply a fact); every unit, including yours, has been getting patients all day (more facts). I need you and three other units each to take a patient" (we're all sharing a heavy load). "If we can get these four patients out of the ED, we can avoid reroute or shutting off the operating rooms" (the consequences: if we can't work this out, with the stress on we, not *me* or *you*).
> *Med-surg nurse to nursing supervisor*: "Well, we're getting slammed too," (a fact) "but we'll do our part. Can you give us a breather after this patient?"

Nursing supervisor: "Absolutely (positive feedback), as long as it doesn't get any worse and we aren't putting patients at risk" (conditional affirmation with the patient coming first).

Simple conversations like these are negotiations, occuring hundreds of times a day in your organization. Investing in negotiation skills for your staff is an extremely important concept for you as a leader. It involves three simple steps, augmented by six negotiation tools.

Negotiation Steps
1. Discovering your expectations
2. Discovering their expectations
3. Negotiating expectations for inventing options for mutual gain

Negotiation Tools
1. Empowerment
2. Point-of-impact intervention
3. Service recovery
4. Dealing with difficult patients
5. Dealing with B-team members
6. Dealing with B-team bosses

You and your staff need to know each of these steps and be skilled at using all six tools, depending on the needs of the situation. Let's look at each of the steps and tools.

NEGOTIATION STEP 1: DISCOVERING EXPECTATIONS—YOURS

In a customer service text, it may seem curious to start by discovering your expectations instead of starting with the patient. However, it is important for you and your staff to recognize that everyone approaches each healthcare encounter with expectations of their own. As we saw in Chapter 2, the first source of expectation is from answering the question, "Is this a patient or is this a customer?" But staff have other expectations as well. What are their expectations for this specific clinical encounter, what percent patient or percent customer are they facing? They need to ask themselves, *Is this really the right patient for me, for this unit, for this segment of healthcare?* Just as you probably think about the negotiation strategy you will use when you enter a meeting, your staff must also think of negotiation strategies regarding their expectations for the clinical encounters that they have.

Distress, Eustress, and the Stress Tolerance Level

In addition to assessing expectations for the next meeting, the next negotiation, or the next patient, staff also would be wise to assess where they are on their own stress tolerance curve (a concept we learned from a friend and colleague, Joan Kyes, RN). We tend to think of stress as bad, but not all stress is truly negative, as Hans Selye (1978) demonstrated in his research nearly 30 years ago. It takes a certain amount of stress—positive stress, called "eustress" in Selye's model—to motivate us, to get us out of bed in the morning, to move us forward in our careers, to get us to pursue further education, to get us to go to the "nth" meeting of the day, to meet with the disgruntled medical staff member or employee. It is only when stress reaches, in Malcom Gladwell's phrase, "the tipping point"— when it goes over the top and becomes *distress*—that it assumes the characteristic of negative stress, the more common meaning of the term *stress* (Gladwell 2002). That's the point at which we reach our stress tolerance level, or STL. The question then becomes, "Are you capable of the self-knowledge and self-reflection required to understand what you look like, what you feel like, as you approach the limits of your STL?" For example, how do you feel, what are the warning signals, when you think to yourself, *If one more person with one more problem or one more complaint comes whining to me, I'm going to …*

… scream, yell, cry, jump out the window, choke them—whatever your response is to distress or negative stress.

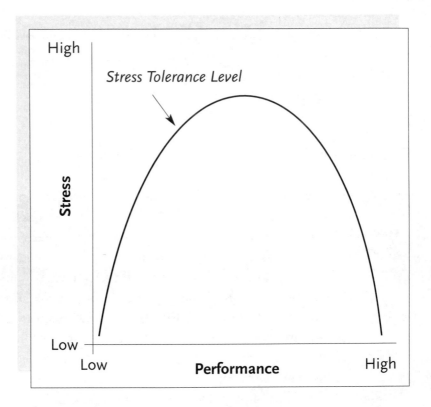

Train yourself to know when you're reaching your STL. Does your pulse go up, your face blush, your stomach churn, your palms sweat? Whatever it is that you look like and feel like—and it is different for each individual—figure it out ahead of time so you'll know your profile as you approach your STL (and before anyone else does).

What do you do when you are approaching your STL? Decompress, de-stress, take a time out, close the door, turn off the lights, lay on the floor, put on some music, think pleasant thoughts, look at a picture of your family—whatever is needed to step back from the precipice of your STL. Again, it varies for each individual, but you should know what it takes to rebuild your reservoir of stress acceptance, to come back down to the left side of the curve. Don't take on the next challenge facing you—whether it is a tough negotiation as a healthcare leader or a tough patient or family with high expectations for a caregiver—without de-stressing, to the best extent possible, prior to entering the negotiation.

Disconnect Your Hot Buttons

Everyone has hot buttons. Not everyone knows what they are. If you don't know what your hot buttons are, ask your staff—they know. Are you familiar with 360° feedback? Think of this as a mini version. If you're really ready for a hot-button reality check, ask your spouse or significant other, and especially your children—they *really* know how to push your buttons. It's important to recognize what your hot buttons are prior to negotiating expectations.

After introspection and "mini 360°" feedback, you know what your hot buttons are—now disconnect them. Mentally, put yourself in an encounter where your hot buttons would normally be pushed: dealing with a particularly troublesome direct report or department manager, speaking with the shrill family member of an unhappy patient, or perhaps simply going into the room of an unhappy patient. Imagine your response as your hot buttons are pushed—the negative, nonproductive ways in which you fail to invent options for mutual gain.

Now "rewind" and take the scenario back to the start. Mentally envision the stress of the hot button situation—but this time, envision yourself not reacting in your normal hot-button way. See yourself handling the situation gracefully, hear the charm and dignity in your voice as you decompress this difficult situation, and feel how relaxed you are as the negotiation unfolds with equanimity. You've disconnected your hot button. You've learned, mentally, how to handle the situation differently. Now do it for all the rest of your hot buttons.

NEGOTIATION STEP 2: DISCOVERING EXPECTATIONS—THEIRS

How can you discover the expectations of those with whom you negotiate—whether they are your colleagues, the medical staff, or patients? Two simple words suffice: Ask them.

The vast majority of the time, a straightforward, nonconfrontational question—*What are your expectations?*—gets a straightforward, nonconfrontational answer. While we sometimes need to help others discover their expectations with a series of nearly Socratic questions (What would success look like to you in this project? How can we best take into account our employee's expectations? How would you like me to handle your concerns?), we can usually clarify expectations fairly simply. Nonetheless, *how* we ask can be a source of interest, particularly in clinical encounters.

- *Emergency physician to patient*: "What's wrong with you?"
  Patient to emergency physician: "You're the doctor, you're supposed to know, that's why I came here."
- *Healthcare provider to patient*: "What brings you here today?"
  Patient to healthcare provider: "The bus."

I once picked up an ED chart and astutely read the nurses' note—why not take advantage of our nursing colleagues' insights on the patient prior to going in the room?—which read, "Patient states he fell out of a tree."

Walking in the room, I extended my hand and, with a warm smile, said, "Mr. Smith, I'm Dr. Mayer. I'm the emergency physician who will be caring for you today. I understand from the nurses' note that you fell out of a tree. What did you hit when you landed?"

He replied, "The ground, Newton!"

That incident happened over 15 years ago, but it taught me to be a little clearer in my questions regarding expectations. (Incidentally, after considerable reflection on this matter, I don't think it was the "the ground" that bothered me—I think it was "Newton!" Clearly, this was an educated man who understood the laws of physics. After all, he didn't say, "Einstein" or "Dumbo," he said "Newton!") Notwithstanding that little bon mot, I have found it best to negotiate from a clear understanding of the patient's expectation by asking simple questions such as, "What are your expectations?" or "How can I help you?"

Restate Expectations

To obtain the maximum clarity regarding expectations, it is wise to restate the expectations in simple, clear language after you have heard them.

- *CEO to department director*: "What I heard you say is that your department is different and therefore shouldn't be held to the same service excellence standards as the rest of the team. Did I hear you correctly?"
- *Lab director to vice president of medical affairs*: "Okay, it is my understanding that 'success' in this matter means that 95 percent of STAT laboratory requests will be completed in 20 minutes or less? Is that correct?"
- *Chief nurse executive to nursing managers*: "I heard you say that nurse recruitment and retention would improve dramatically if we could deliver on a commitment to no more than four patients at any one time for any medical-surgical nurse. Is that correct?"

These examples help you to understand how restating expectations can help ensure clarity in negotiation of expectations.

NEGOTIATION STEP 3: INVENT OPTIONS FOR MUTUAL GAIN

Once you have a clear sense of your expectations in the service encounter and you have also discovered the patient, family, or staff expectations, you need to assess ways in which these expectations differ, since this is the point from which negotiations will proceed. For example, in the "Are they patients or are they customers" exercise, we found that the lady with a heart attack was, in the healthcare workers' estimation, a patient. Here, then is the question: *Does she agree with you?*

The answer is "Yes" because the sicker she is, the more horizontal she is, and the more likely she (and her family) is to agree with your customer service diagnosis. This is an example where expectations are likely similar or congruous, and less negotiation is needed.

But what about the three-year-old child at 3 a.m. with the fever? Do the parents agree that their child is more of a customer, or more vertical? Absolutely not. Clearly they think the child is a patient, nearly horizontal. Now it becomes a situation that involves negotiation.

Obviously, telling the parents they have unreasonable expectations isn't going to work. Nor is saying any of the following (all of which are drawn from real conservations with patients):

- "You're not the sickest patient here."
- "This isn't really a fever."
- "What are you wasting my time for?"
- "You came to the emergency department for *this*?"

This not only doesn't work, it makes the situation much worse. So does the following comment, made in response to a patient who said to his nurse, "But I'm in pain!" Her reply? "Honey, we're *all* in pain here."

Instead, use the *inventing options for mutual gain* concept. Here are some examples of how combining communication skills and inventing options for mutual gain can work.

Patient/Family/Staff	Inventing Options for Mutual Gain
"But I'm in pain—can't you give me something to take it away?"	"We expect you to have some pain in the postoperative period, particularly on the first day. But your patient-controlled anesthesia pump is designed to give you control of your pain without giving you too much medication."
"What did my CT scan show?"	"Your doctor is seeing patients in the office. Let me see if she or her nurse (or nurse practitioner or physician's aide) can talk to the radiologist and let you know before she comes by on rounds this evening."
"I have to wait for the specialist?"	"We think your case requires the input of a specialist in this area. But I'll check to see when she's coming and make sure all the data are ready and available. Is there anything else I can do to help?"
"I can't go home from the hospital until 6 p.m. I don't have a ride and my family is at work."	"I've arranged for you to be cared for in our Discharge Lounge while you wait for your family. You'll be more comfortable there."
"It's unreasonable to hold our unit to service standards when we're so short staffed."	[As the CEO] "Both staffing and service excellence are core competencies I expect from our leaders. We can track satisfaction scores by provider to assess agency versus permanent staff. Most important is to remember that the number one reason for service excellence is that it makes all our jobs easier, not harder!"

Now that we've addressed the three steps in negotiation, let's go into the toolbox to look at the skills necessary to negotiate effectively.

NEGOTIATION TOOL 1: EMPOWERMENT

Empowerment. Great word. Great concept. Yet often overused and misunderstood. Tom Peters called it "controlled chaos" and "the great energy liberator." But what does it have to do with negotiation?

Empowerment is the sustained and deep commitment to a philosophy that well-selected, well-trained staff are our biggest resource and they deserve to have the authority to make reasonably appropriate decisions over the span of influence for which they are held accountable. To empower your staff, simply enact a policy today that states, *make no decisions at a higher level that can be made at a lower level.*

As we've stated repeatedly, healthcare is a personal service business. The unit of transaction is always a person. It's not a chest x-ray or a coronary artery bypass and graft or a bronchoscopy. It's all of these—and many more—done *by* people *for* patients. The people responsible for the service delivery must be entrusted with the power to make service meaningful. That doesn't mean that there aren't appropriate checks and supervision; it means that staff should be able to make their own decisions when appropriate. Too often in healthcare, however, we are told that "When it comes to empowerment, the words and the music just don't match."

At one prestigious medical center with a reputation for having empowered programs, we asked a large audience of employees a simple question: "Are you empowered?" The silence, frankly, was a bit disquieting, until a small voice from the last row said, "They *tell* us we are." You tell your staff they are empowered, but where's the substance, and how do you give it to them? Often in healthcare, the words (empowerment) and the music (empowerment in action) don't match.

Thick-Rule-Book Organizations Versus Thin-Rule-Book Organizations

Healthcare organizations who deliver true service excellence understand that service doesn't reside in a customer service manual, in a service department, or in a thick rule book that explains every detail of how to act, how to dress, what to say, what to do, what not to do. Greatness in service comes from thin rule books, not thick ones. Thick-rule-book organizations delineate everything and every way in which service is to be delivered and insist on adherence. Thin-rule-book organizations create the broad and important mission and vision regarding service and the organizations' commitment to it, but they rely on leadership and management to act as catalysts to help employees discover, uncover, and create service excellence in ways that they know better than you ever could. Indeed, as we discuss "creating moments of truth" in the next chapter, it is wise to remember that it is *better to have one person practicing empowered customer service than a hundred posted mission statements proclaiming it.*

Make your commitment to service excellence clear, but keep a thin rule book—then turn your staff loose to create that service. Celebrate service success stories and reward your champions, and A-team behaviors (invented by them, not you) will flourish.

Narrow Corridors for Success, or Wide Corridors for Success?

Service excellence occurs in organizations that not only have thin rule books but also wide corridors for success. There are many ways in which to succeed in service—not just "the boss's way" or "the company's way." If your organization is one in which you hear the familiar quote, "My way or the highway," you can be certain that neither empowerment nor service excellence will occur. Hire right (as we will discuss in the next chapter), train them well, give them servant leaders who exemplify the service ethic, and then turn them loose. They will create more than a leadership team could ever possibly imagine, as the next chapter illustrates.

NEGOTIATION TOOL 2: POINT-OF-IMPACT INTERVENTION

After studying patient complaints and concerns carefully for over ten years, we found an important fact: Over 95 percent of the time, the caregivers realized there was a problem or potential problem *at the time the patient's care was delivered.*

Point-of-Impact Skills

For that reason, we created point-of-impact intervention as the intersection of two vectors—empowerment and negotiation skills—to make clear to our staff that they are empowered to solve problems when they occur using negotiation skills. Point-of-impact skills involve the following eight points.

Identify the problem and address it immediately
Let them know that you are aware something has gone wrong and that you want to "fix it." Be clear that you understand that their expectations have not been met.

Establish the fact that you know there has been a breakdown
Use the two most powerful words in the English language: *I'm sorry.* Say it early, and say it often. Make sure the staff uses it liberally. Also use the "blameless apology." The blameless apology simply recognizes the fact that some service standard has been breached, that you apologize for it, but that you do so in a blameless way. For example:

> "I'm sorry it's taken so long to see you, but I'll try to move you through this system as fast as possible from this point on." It *doesn't*

say, "I'm sorry we're turkeys" or "I'm sorry everyone *else* is a turkey" or even "I'm sorry you had to wait, but we couldn't give a flip what time you get seen." It's a sincere apology, but it does not assess blame, as assessing blame at the time of the complaint is usually a waste of time, effort, and energy.

Another example:

"I'm sorry you felt the staff was rude." Did you just say the staff was rude? *No*—simply that you are sorry they felt the staff was rude. Big difference.

Wipe the slate clean

Try to get the proverbial "tabula rasa." Use phrases such as "I know you feel this hasn't gone well up to this point, but let me see if I can help you through this." Here's a story one of our emergency physicians (Dr. Sharon Day) told us:

I was coming on the morning shift and was on sign-out rounds with the night doctor, who was explaining to me that because they had lost the spinal fluid sample on a child in whom they were ruling out meningitis, they had to redo the spinal tap. I saw the father sitting in the room, obviously frustrated, angry, and extremely tired from a long night—and with his child getting not one but two spinal taps. I thought to myself, "We are going to get a seriously angry letter from this guy!" But I put my arm on his shoulder and said, 'Sir, I know you've had a long night and you look really tired. Can I get you a cup of coffee? I'll make sure your son's care goes as fast as it possibly can from this point forward." He took the coffee—and we did get a letter. However, it was a letter of compliment not complaint.

With that one simple act, she wiped a difficult slate clean—and created great service. That's a "two for". She not only killed a complaint, she generated a compliment.

Reestablish their expectations

Our studies (Mayer and Cates 1999; Mayer et al. 1998) indicate that over 90 percent of patient complaints come from an initial failure to clearly establish patient or family expectations. In essence, the wrong customer service diagnosis is made and is therefore being treated incorrectly. Reestablish their expectations, clarify their expectations—then you can treat the *right* customer service diagnosis.

Negotiate and resolve issues

Give your staff the power and authority to "solve it on the spot." Can they give out meal tickets, offer coffee bar courtesies, or write off bills? One system in Michigan hands out movie tickets if the patient waits too long.

When possible, meet their expectations

Talk to them, relieve their pain, answer their questions. Give them specified time frames for follow-up, and use expectation creation to give clearly identified expectations, including time lines, for what and when things will happen.

Offer reasonable alternatives

The customer is *not* always right. Nor are the corollary statements "The customer is not always right, but they are always the customer" or "The customer is not always right, but you have to make them think they're right." None of these bromides are correct. Don't say such nonsense to your staff. Why? Because if the customer is always right, what does that make you? Always wrong! The point is, you can't always meet every expectation, but you can give them reasonable alternatives in language with a strong service orientation.

When all else fails, give them someone else to talk to

Give your staff the ability to defer to leadership and management's strong service commitment. Let them talk to the charge physician, the charge nurse, or the department director. Give them scripts that say, "I'm sorry I haven't been able to resolve all of your concerns and expectations. But service is very important to us here. With your permission, I'll leave a voice mail with my manager and she'll contact you as soon as her schedule allows."

Let staff use the voice mail system to communicate these concerns, and then ensure that leaders and managers are returning calls—preferably within 24 hours. Your managers don't have time to field these calls. Then you don't have much of a service excellence program. Service success requires all leaders and managers, including administrators and CEOs, to be close to the action in service delivery and service recovery. When you return these calls, use service recovery skills, as discussed below.

NEGOTIATION TOOL 3: SERVICE RECOVERY SURVIVAL SKILLS

The best of the writings on service recovery are listed in the "More on This" section at the end of the chapter. We'll give you the mini version.

In other words, *how* you contact them is less important than *how soon* you contact them. The service literature is replete with studies showing that if you identify and resolve a problem within 48 hours of its occurrence, you

In person...
By phone...
By letter...
The sooner the better!

can retain that customer or even turn him or her into a loyal customer. But if your service recovery exceeds 72 hours, you have likely lost any reasonable chance of recovering his or her business. Worse yet, some of them become "crusaders" who will bad mouth your healthcare system at every opportunity—to the community, to their friends and neighbors, in public forums, to your board members, even to the press. Transform crusaders with the preventative skills of point-of-impact intervention. If this misses them, then use the following service recovery skills:

- Listen
- Apologize
- Fix it
- Something extra
- Follow through
- Follow up

Listen

Of all of the communication skills, listening is by far the most important, particularly when a patient/customer feels that his or her expectations have not been met. Most of this listening will be done on the telephone, although some patients and their families will want to come to your office to talk. For the telephone complaints, get a cup of coffee (and in some cases one of those tall, frothy, foamy drinks) and get comfortable—because you are going to be listening for a *long* time to some complaints. Like a child with a tantrum, some complainers simply have to wear themselves out. Let them know at the outset that service is important to you and you would like to know how it can be improved. Take notes and wait until they have had a chance to fully vent their concerns. Use *active listening* to clarify their concerns, using language like, "Mrs. Jones, I appreciate your having brought this matter to my attention. Here's what I heard you say regarding your concerns…" Listening is *the* most important communication skill—develop it in yourself and your staff. The most difficult communication skill is listening effectively, empathetically, and actively.

Apologize

This is an area where many in healthcare have a problem. Make sure your staff knows how to say the two most powerful words in the English language, "I'm sorry." As discussed in the previous chapter, use the blameless apology. You should not be apologizing for your staff, their behavior, lack of staffing, or other issues. You should let patients/customers know that you're sorry that this problem occurred. The following examples are how NOT to apologize:

- "I'm sorry our staff are morons."
- "I'm sorry the doctor was so obnoxious to you and your family."
- "I'm sorry we are so short staffed."
- "We can't find good help!"

Examples of the blameless apology might include:

- "I'm sorry this happened to you."
- "I'm sorry you feel that you were ignored."
- "I'm sorry that we couldn't do a better job in meeting your expectations."
- "I'm sorry you feel that the staff was rude to you."

The old adage is often true—a gentle word does turn away wrath. Many patients have a genuine and legitimate (in their mind) sense of outrage regarding the complaints they have about their experiences with healthcare. As leaders and managers, it is your job to decompress that outrage and to decode it in an attempt to turn it into something positive, particularly when it comes to using complaints to eliminate B-team behaviors and fix your faulty processes.

Fix It

As we indicated in Chapter 1, complaint analysis is one of the most effective tools available to a healthcare leader. Using service failures as a guide toward improving A-team behaviors; eliminating B-team behaviors; and empowering staff through feedback, training, and improved processes is essential. Not all complainers are nut cases. As Mark Twain said, "Nothing defines us better than how we behave toward fools." We are certainly not implying that patients who have complaints are fools—far from it. Their insights into how service appears to them can often be gifts that allow you to see yourselves in a light that truly helps you improve services, processes, and outcomes.

But you should pay particular attention when you are handling what you consider to be "unreasonable" expectations.

Not only should you "fix it" in service recovery, you also need to let the patient know that you have used his or her concerns in a positive fashion as a part of process improvement. A simple statement like, "I appreciate your letting me know about your concerns, as we can only improve our service when people are as kind as you have been in informing us about those concerns" lets them know you appreciate their feedback and take their concerns seriously.

Something Extra

Several years ago, we handled what at the time seemed to be the "complainer from hell." This gentleman was concerned about the care provided to his daughter (as is often the case, people are usually more distressed about the care provided to their family members than that provided to themselves). This gentleman started outraged, stayed outraged, and became more outraged through the course of our attempts at service recovery. As with many complaints, what set him off had some substance to it—in this case a medical staff member failing to arrive in the emergency department in a timely fashion. It was compounded by further B-team behaviors on the part of this medical staff specialist. Although this specialist did not work for us, we understood that it is important to take the approach of "owning the complaint" and being the guide back to service success. Our philosophy is that whoever identifies the complaint owns the complaint and acts as a guide through the recovery process, including telephone calls, letters, and follow-up to be sure that the problem has been addressed. To take such an approach, these are the sorts of questions you engender in your organization:

- "Who owns the problem?"
- "How did you guide him or her back to service success?"

In this particular case, it seemed as if *nothing* would please this gentleman or turn away his wrath. Multiple phone calls and communications went back and forth over a period of several weeks. Finally, we sent him a letter that read, in part:

> Thank you for taking time from your busy schedule to inform us of your concerns in rich detail, so that we could appropriately address them. Please accept the enclosed gift certificate to Outback Steakhouse as a symbol of our appreciation for the time you took to help us improve our service.

Now, you (or your management team) might say, "There is *no way* that a simple $25 Outback Steakhouse coupon is going to make this problem go away!" But in fact it did—we got a very complimentary letter back from this gentleman, thanking us and indicating that he would certainly use our services if he needed emergency care for his family in the future. We turned a complainer into a loyal customer. Think about the following: How many doctors do you have on your staff who have both a Jaguar and a Mercedes, yet they would trample each other to get to the drug representative for a free plastic pen? What do you think they would do to get an Outback Steakhouse coupon?

Everybody loves a gift. Judiciously and appropriately utilized, "something extra" can be helpful to put service recovery into a different perspective. Meal tickets, gift certificates, flowers, fruit baskets—use your imagination and empower your staff to give them as well. However, such gifts usually need to be restricted to service problems, as opposed to technical problems. If a patient or family is judged to be potentially litigious, either by your estimation or that from the risk management people, gifts can be considered offensive or an attempt to "buy off" potential litigants. Notwithstanding such circumstances, for service problems, allowing your managers to use "something extra" in service recovery can be extremely helpful. Whether it is free meals, free parking, or certificates for the coffee bar in the atrium, this is an important part of service recovery.

Follow Through, Follow Up

When a patient takes the time to identify a problem and you agree that indeed a behavior, process, or system needs to be fixed, fix it! Assuring patients that you have followed through on their concerns to not only fix the problem but also made sure that it stays fixed is an extremely important part of service recovery. This is important not just to the patient but to your staff as well. If you are serious about complaint management as a way of improving service recovery and eliminating B-team behaviors and processes, there must be demonstrable evidence that there has been appropriate follow-up and follow-through. In your letters to the patient/customer, reassure them that this follow-through has occurred.

NEGOTIATION TOOL 4: DEALING WITH THE DIFFICULT PATIENT

Dealing with difficult patients—some would say "B-team patients"—is a tool that you and each member of your staff will need. While similar to service recovery, dealing with difficult patients is done in "real time," preferably at the bedside. As mentioned previously, the most important skill, both here and in service recovery, is listening actively, empathetically, and compassionately. Say "I'm sorry," but do so in a blameless way.

Learning How to Say You Are Sorry

Note that none of these following sentences apportion blame; they simply acknowledge the patient or family's concerns and indicate you're sorry they feel that way.

- "I'm sorry you feel the staff wasn't listening to you."

- "I'm sorry you feel the doctor didn't communicate well with your father."
- "I'm sorry you feel we've failed to meet your expectations."

"What Can I Do to Make This Right for You?"

This question may seem like a time bomb, bad advice, or a risk-management nightmare. However, if you and your staff have learned the blameless apology and how to say you are sorry without acknowledging fault or wrong, over 90 percent of patients or families who have a complaint who are asked, "What can I do to make this right for you?" have the same response:

"I just don't want it to happen to anyone else."

When they say this, a great response is, "Thank you for letting us know about this issue. I assure you I will follow up and make changes to keep this from happening again."

The Power of "I" and the Elusiveness of "We" and "They"

Much of the language of healthcare has a vaguely elusive nature about it. Think about how many times you hear questions being answered with these responses:

- "Not to my knowledge."
- "Not that I'm aware of."
- "Not that I know with the data available at the present time."

Small wonder that patients and families find this confusing, if not evasive. Similarly, notice how we talk about complaints using "they" most often and less commonly "we."

- "The staff tells me they didn't lose your valuables."
- "The lab lost your blood sample. They do that all the time."
- "We can't be expected to meet noncritical needs or expectations. After all, we're a hospital, not a four-star hotel."

This sort of language angers normal people—and infuriates B-team/difficult patients. Instead, use the first person singular whenever you can.

- "I'm sorry this happened, but I'll take care of it."
- "I apologize to you and your family. I'll look into it and contact you within 48 hours."
- "I'll make the appropriate changes to see this doesn't happen again."

Use the Volume Control

Difficult patients and families tend to operate at extraordinarily high volume, since they are angry, frustrated, and seemingly at the end of their rope. The louder, more obnoxious, and more unreasonable they are, the softer, more quiet, and more reasonable you should become. Dialing your volume down as their's goes up helps de-escalate the problem.

Use Proactive Body Language

When people are angry with you, they tend to point, gesticulate, and step forward. Use the power of your body language to a positive, proactive effect. Instead of crossing your arms in a closed, negative posture, open your hands, arms, and facial expression to indicate concern, sympathy, empathy, and openness.

Remember: You Are Onstage

The Disney Corporation uses the onstage-offstage analogy to emphasize the performance aspect of service to their "cast members." By not calling them employees, staff are reminded that they should always remain "in character" when they are "onstage" in front of the public. The problem in healthcare is that you are *always* onstage, except perhaps when you are off-duty in the staff lounge or in the office with the door closed. Most of your staff will encounter angry patients and their families either at the bedside or at the nursing station. Help them to understand that this is onstage, in that other patients, families, and their fellow healthcare workers are observing the interaction. Use the onstage concept to recruit allies by being unfailingly professional, calm, courteous, and compassionate—even in the face of anger and resentment. We have received many letters, voice mails, and e-mails that began, "I want to compliment your staff for being highly professional in a difficult situation I witnessed…"

Take the Sail Out of Their Wind

The old adage "Take the wind out of their sails" is unfortunately inaccurate. After all, the complaining patients or family have a seemingly inexhaustible wind supply. Their wind is precisely the problem. Instead, take the *sail* out of their *wind*. In other words, don't give them anything to blow *against*. If there is no resistance to the wind, the ship won't move off course when those ill winds blow. How do we take the sail out of their wind? Try the following steps:

- *Don't interrupt.* If you ask patients, they'll tell you that healthcare staff are notorious for interrupting patients' responses to the questions they are asked. On average, a nurse interrupts after 1 minute and 14 seconds, while doctors interrupt after only 48 seconds. Whenever possible, let them finish their story.

- *Don't resist.* This is usually not the time to confront them with the facts. When they say they waited 1 hour and 48 minutes for a chest x-ray and you total the time and say it was "only" 1 hour and 37 minutes, it doesn't help. Let them "win" on the small points, so you can concentrate on the big ones.
- *Focus on their concerns.* As patients tell their stories about their journey through healthcare, they almost always provide a certain amount of extraneous detail. Sift through these details to focus on their areas of concern.
- *Focus on expectations.* Ask patients and family members how the hospital failed to meet their expectations. Many patients are seemingly angry about everything, particularly if they feel their dignity has been offended. Help them focus their expectations.
- *Do your homework.* Whenever possible, review the chart and speak to the healthcare workers involved in their care for their perspective on the encounter. Doing your homework up front saves time in future meetings.
- *Come to closure.* By doing your homework, preparing carefully, and listening empathetically and skillfully, you should be able to resolve complaints at the initial meeting in the majority of cases. Restate the patient/family concerns, express an apology, and state an action plan for follow-up if needed. Send a note of closure, along with a business card, to the patient.

NEGOTIATION TOOL 5: DEALING WITH B-TEAM MEMBERS

One of the questions we are asked most often is, "How do I deal with the B-team members? How can I get them to move to the A-team?"

As we said at the outset of the book, two fundamental truths must be kept in mind when any change in human behavior is sought:

1. All meaningful and lasting change is intrinsically, not extrinsically, motivated
2. The #1 reason to focus on service excellence is that it makes the job easier.

Trying to get someone to change for *your* reasons is virtually condemned to failure. Doing it "because the boss, or anyone else, says so" has been a mantra for leadership failure. Why? Because people fundamentally need to be shown that it is better *for them* to change than to continue in their old habits. There has to be not only a wedge, a driving force to move them away from their old behavior, but also a magnet, a force that pulls them toward a better way of doing things (i.e., it makes the job easier). So we need to begin with a clear understanding of this psychological insight and show them both the wedge—the B-team behavior—and the magnet—the A-team behavior that makes their job easier. The process looks like this: *Be proactive, not reactive.*

Don't wait for the B-team behavior to rear its ugly head; be positive and proactive in promoting service excellence and the A-team behaviors. Accentuate and celebrate compliments, showing how A-team behaviors work and how they are rewarded. Give the magnet of A-team behaviors meaning.

Solicit Team Input

One of the questions leaders face is, "Is this person's behavior my problem?" Confidentially and professionally, seek the view of key members of the team regarding the B-team member and his or her behavior. Hold this information in strict confidence, but use it to ensure you have an accurate sense of the disruption the B-team member creates. Then use the following steps to eliminate the disruption.

Tie the Effects of the B-Team Behavior to the Team

Many leaders and managers make counseling of B-team members personal: "I want you to do this…" or "I don't want you to do that…" It is usually better to tie the negative impact of the B-team behavior to its impact on the team and its vision, mission, and strategies. (Of course, it is always gratifying to say, "Exactly how did your kicking this patient in the groin fit in with the team's customer service initiative?")

Given that the team vision, mission, and strategy are mutually developed and agreed on, relating B-team actions to those team goals can be helpful and keeps any discussion from becoming personal. It will also, if done correctly, encourage the B-team member to improve his or her performance to better reflect the team's vision, mission, and strategy. Because it has not been made "personal," he or she will be more motivated to improve.

Reflect, Write It Down, then Act Quickly

Don't let anger or frustration at what often seems like frequent—or even recalcitrant—B-team behaviors cause you to react out of that anger and frustration. Instead, reflect on what the B-team member has done, the effect on the rest of the team, and the context in which it has occurred. Take the time to write it down—including what happened, its downstream effects, possible course of action, team input—and then decide what to do. It may sound odd, but it is usually a good idea to outline what you are going to say, how you are going to say it, what reaction to expect, and how to respond to those reactions. However, once you've done this—and it shouldn't take more than 24 to 72 hours—act quickly and decisively, with a clear plan of action. Finally, no one likes to be the bearer of bad tidings (well, some people do, but that's another topic altogether), so don't put it off. As soon as you know what needs to be said and how to say it—say it.

Be Specific

Too often, leaders counsel others in language that is, at best, imprecise and, at worst, unclear and passive: "Gee, it would be great if you would, maybe, you know, do things just a little bit differently—if you don't mind." Don't do that. Be clear, be concise, and be specific. We like this format: "When you do x, it results in y; try z instead."

Think about this for a moment. What is x? Clearly, it is the B-team behavior about which you should give clear and precise detail. What's y? Well, y is the result, the negative effect of the B-team behavior, whether that is patient complaints, family concerns, disruptiveness to the other staff, risk management concerns, poor morale, etc. How about z—what's that? Clearly, z is the A-team behavior you recommend, a concrete example of how it could be done and the improved effect that results.

Give Them a Mentor

All of you have doctors, nurses, laboratory technicians, radiology technicians, and department directors who are widely respected and admired. Some, perhaps with no formal leadership position, are just great people to have in the organization. Others admire, respect, and look up to them as role models. Use these A-team members in your organization as mentors to the B-team members. They can have a profound and dramatic effect on your B-team members by showing them there is a better, and easier, way of doing things. These A-team members can show them the magnet A-team behaviors and habits that make the job easier.

Celebrate Success

When the B-team members start exhibiting A-team behaviors, it's time to break out the champagne (figuratively, at best) and celebrate. When they start getting compliments, make sure there is a public celebration of the A-team behavior from the B-team member. This is very powerful stuff, and a symbol of hope to others. When the most egregious of the B-team members start behaving differently, people take serious notice. There is also the Machiavellian aspect that the service excellence change is exponentially accelerated when Nurse Ratched, Dr. Torquemada, and Administrator Scrooge start getting compliments.

Be Prepared for Failure—Fire Right

Some staff members don't get it and will never get it. It doesn't mean they are bad people. However, it does often mean they need to be in a different job (i.e., the "deep joy, deep need" theory) or out of healthcare entirely. As the old saying goes, "Some people you don't get even with, but away from." Don't get us wrong—it's never enjoyable to fire or transfer an employee or colleague, but sometimes it is necessary. Although some B-team members need the remedial course in customer service—they need to go back for additional study, counseling, and homework—others simply do not have the servant's heart that is a requirement to be successful in healthcare.

NEGOTIATION TOOL 6: DEALING WITH B-TEAM BOSSES

Sometimes—not infrequently—the revolution comes from within. What do you do if the troops are fired up for customer service, but the department director or assistant administrator is not? Happily, customer service is one of those areas where it is better to ask for forgiveness than permission. If you have staff who want to cultivate ideas for customer service, but managers who are an obstacle, there are ways to cultivate creativity without mutiny.

First, reach down in the organization, not to meddle or micromanage but to be clear that service excellence is an organizational passion, not a departmental initiative. Leadership team meetings should emphasize this, as well as stressing that you want to hear creative ideas and success stories from throughout the organization. Second, be aware and tolerant that managers are of necessity and by nature at different stages in their learning curves regarding service excellence. Many of them need their own mentors when it comes to nurturing and encouraging A-team behaviors. Third, we cannot overemphasize the importance of being visible, vocal, and unceasing in your commitment to service. Making service rounds in the patient care areas and asking patients, "How can we do this better?" to develop as clear an understanding as possible of how the service is delivered is essential to permeating the organization with a commitment to service. Your time is very valuable, but it is never better spent than seeing and being seen by the patients and the staff who serve them. Fourth, just as you encourage your staff to be specific with B-team employees, so should you be with your leadership team. The "When you do *x*..." model is a good one for leaders as well as employees.

Finally, as we'll discuss in the next chapter, it is critical that you hire right when you select members of your management team. Ask potential department directors and assistant/associate administrators open-ended yet penetrating questions about their commitment to service excellence, including examples of how they've handled difficult service problems well and references you can contact regarding their commitment to service. They'll get the message: In this organization, service is essential!

SURVIVAL SKILLS SUMMARY

- Negotiation skills are essential in healthcare, not just for the management team but for every employee.
- Despite negotiation being a core competency in healthcare, very little training has been provided in this skill.
- Because there is frequently a difference between our expectations and the patient's expectations, we need to help our staff learn to negotiate more effectively.
- Use the "inventing options for mutual gain" exercise to help your staff understand the crucial role of successful negotiation.
- The second Survival Skill is negotiating agreement and resolution of expectations and includes three negotiation steps and six negotiation tools:

Negotiation Steps
1. Discovering your expectations
2. Discovering their expectations
3. Negotiating expectations by inventing options for mutual gain

Negotiation Tools
1. Empowerment
2. Point-of-impact intervention
3. Service recovery
4. Dealing with difficult patients
5. Dealing with B-team members
6. Dealing with B-team bosses

REFERENCES

Gladwell, M. 2002. *The Tipping Point: How Little Things Can Make a Big Difference.* San Francisco: Back Bay Books.

Mayer, T., and R. J. Cates. 1999. "Service Excellence in Health Care." *Journal of the American Medical Association* 282 (13): 1281–83.

Mayer, T. A., R. J. Cates, M. J. Mastorovich, and D. L. Royalty. 1998. "Emergency Department Patient Satisfaction: Customer Service Training Improves Patient Satisfaction and Ratings of Physician and Nurse Skill." *Journal of Healthcare Management* 43 (5): 427–40.

Seyle, H. 1978. *The Stress of Life*. New York: McGraw-Hill.

MORE ON THIS

The best of the books on negotiation, all of which are very practical.

Fisher, R., W. Ury, and B. Patton. 1991. *Getting to Yes: Negotiating Agreement Without Giving In*, 2nd ed. New York: Penguin.

Ury, W. 1999. *Getting to Peace: Transforming Conflict at Home, at Work, and in the World*. New York: Penguin.

———. 1993. *Getting Past No: Negotiating Your Way from Confrontation to Cooperation*. New York: Bantam,

Each of these books is excellent and contains good sections on service recovery.

Frieberg, K., and J. Frieberg. 1997. *Nuts! Southwest Airlines' Crazy Recipe for Business and Personal Success*. New York: Broadway Books.

Gitomer, J. 1998. *Customer Satisfaction is Worthless: Customer Loyalty is Priceless*. Austin, TX: Bard Press.

CHAPTER 5

The Third Survival Skill:
Creating Moments of Truth

THE IDEA OF "moments of truth" is not our invention; indeed, many have claimed the concept as their own. We believe the original description came from Jan Carlzon's 1987 book, *Moments of Truth*. Carlzon was the former CEO of Scandinavian Airways, who assumed that position at the age of 39, at a time when the airline was in serious trouble on all fronts. In resuscitating the airline's reputation for service excellence, he addressed the employees in the following (paraphrased) way:

> You, the employees of Scandinavian Airways, have been defining the airlines as a certain number and types of planes, with specified revenue capacity, specified load capacity, taking off and landing on time, with the passengers' bags getting to the right place.
>
> I don't believe that that's the way that the airway is actually defined. I believe that the airline is defined by 50,000 Moments of Truth a day. A Moment of Truth occurs when you—the employees of Scandinavian Airways—have contact with those we serve—the people who fly the airlines and their friends and family. Thus,

each of you defines the airline on a daily basis by these 50,000 Moments of Truth.

In Carlzon's definition, a moment of truth occurs whenever service employees have an encounter with those they serve. So what? What's the implication for healthcare? After defining moments of truth in Carlzon's fashion, address your staff with a question: "Do you think our patients have any idea how many beds we have in this institution? How many nurses we have? How many doctors? How many cardiovascular surgeons? No. Of course not, but they know you."

Carlzon's message is as simple as this: *From the customers' perspective, the people performing the service are the company.*

MISSION AND VISION

The patients/customers in your healthcare system can't know you or even your leadership and management team to any substantial degree. But they do know those on the front lines—and they will judge *your* service by *their* service. If those on the front line create positive moments of truth (through A-team behaviors), your institution will have a great reputation for service in the community. This starts with your staff understanding the importance of A-team behaviors versus B-team behaviors and continues with them understanding and embracing their role as service providers. They must be servant leaders, as described by Robert Greenleaf (see the "More on This" list at the end of the chapter). They must have a servant's heart; they must know that a part of their deep joy is in meeting the deep needs of others, particularly at the patients' and families' most desperate times. But these people must also know how important service is to you, as a leader of the institution. That importance undoubtedly is reflected in your institution's mission and vision statements. But is that matched by walking the walk, not just talking the talk?

A word of caution here. It is our view that mission statements must be direct, simple, and easily remembered. Too often these statements drone on and lack "punch." If you can't say it in 30 seconds and the person you're saying it to can't repeat it back in 15 seconds, it's too long and complicated. What's the mission statement in our shop?

**Inova Fairfax Hospital
Emergency Department**

Our goal is to offer our patients
the best patient care and customer service
of any emergency department in the country.

Simple. Clear. Easily remembered. Posted in every room of our emergency department. Easy to deliver on? Hardly. But at least every one of our team members has a clear sense of why we are there. Who designed this mission statement? Our entire emergency department staff participated, since it had to be *their* mission statement, not ours. Remember the old saying, "If they are not with you on the takeoff, they won't be with you on the landing." Give staff a hand in designing their own mission statement, and they are far more likely to embrace it.

Another example is the credo of our company, BestPractices, Incorporated, that provides physician staffing and leadership to hospitals across the country. Everything we do is measured against how well it serves these needs. In our company, if it doesn't serve these needs, it doesn't add value. The third part of the credo is critical; it is easy to have a

---

BestPractices is dedicated to:

• The **SCIENCE** of Clinical Excellence
• The **ART** of Customer Service
• The **BUSINESS** of Execution

---

good idea, but only world-class organizations and great leaders can execute the idea.

It is also important to remember that it is not the mission statement on the wall but the service in the institution that is important. As we said in the previous chapter, *better to have one person practicing empowered customer service than a hundred posted mission statements proclaiming it.*

In our emergency department, we have had the pleasure of working with many customer service champions, including doctors, nurses, administrators, and essential services staff. But three stand out dramatically: Felicia, Fannie, and Bernardo. Felicia and Fannie are runners who take radiology films from the emergency department to the radiologists to be read, after which they return them to the emergency department. Bernardo works in housekeeping. By the measuring stick of years of formal education, they may have the least in our department. But from the benchmark of customer service, they are at the top of the heap. They are unfailingly pleasant, kind, thoughtful, and generous—not just to the patients but to their teammates as well. They have the quintessential servant's heart. When they are on duty, everyone is a little happier, regardless of how high the volume, acuity, or stress levels may be. They exemplify the A-team. What's the point? You've got people just like them in your hospital. Make sure you and your managers know who they are. Turn your Bernardos, Felicias, and Fannies loose, and others will follow them. Celebrate their success and reward your service champions.

It is important to remember that service excellence is elusive in that it is impermanent, is evanescent, and doesn't outlast the encounter. Like fitness or conditioning, it can't be achieved and then have victory declared. It has to occur every day, every night, in every unit throughout your institution, and it must be re-earned each morning when the sun rises. Service 24/7/365 must be your goal. That's hard, because the battle is never over, it's always anew. In service excellence, there is no finish line—the victory is in the running.

MOMENTS OF TRUTH—THE NORDSTROM STORY

Without question, Nordstrom is one of the world's leaders in the retail industry. Its reputation is widely known and, in the estimation of many, justly deserved. Its service successes are detailed in at least two books, *The Nordstrom Way,* by Robert Spector and Patrick McCarthy, and *Fabled Service,* by Betsy Sanders. Betsy Sanders rose up through the ranks of the Nordstrom organization, eventually becoming a motivational speaker on the principles she learned at that company, as detailed in her book (see "More on This" at the end of the chapter). The book is so good that we actually bought it by the case for our emergency department staff when we began our service excellence journey. But the problem with service is that it isn't permanent and it is always unique to the encounter of the individual. Service isn't something you can get right after which you declare victory and leave the playing field. It must be performed every day, by every individual, in every personal circumstance, at every level of the organization.

To illustrate that concept, here's a story that we tell at our seminars. We invite you to share it with others.

When we first began teaching these courses, my oldest daughter, Beth, decided that I needed to look a bit spiffier if I was going to be speaking to sophisticates such as yourselves. At the time, Beth worked for an insurance company, the executives of which were as sharply dressed as you would imagine.

So Beth said, "Dad, you need to go and get a really nice suit where our executives shop—Nordstrom." At the time, I was getting my clothes from a very nice store called Britches (since closed), but the store leaned a little more towards sport coats and casual slacks than finely tailored suits. In fact, the Britches pants I was wearing at the time were not to Beth's liking—she said they were too big and too baggy and they looked like clown pants. Those pants might have looked good on a younger man, a taller man, a thinner man, a more athletic man (some kind of man Dad was not) but to Beth they looked like clown pants. So she said, "Go to Nordstrom, get a new suit, and you'll look great!"

So I went to Nordstrom, dressed fairly casually, where a salesman, Mr. Smith (not his real name), greeted me and began to assist. I told him three things I ordinarily don't say to anyone. First, I told him I was a doctor. I usually don't do that, but I thought he might think that I had some discretionary income and might actually be able to afford a Nordstrom suit. Second, I told him that I taught customer service courses—I thought that would really help me get the best of Nordstrom's service. Third, I told him I had never been to Nordstrom before, so here was a chance for him to capture a customer for life with the legendary Nordstrom's service. I thought that was the trifecta—I couldn't lose with those three things going for me. I thought wrong.

Mr. Smith pulled out a beautiful gray suit and said, "Try this nice gray one on—this is a style the executives in this area are very pleased with." I put the suit on and, indeed, it did look nice, but when Mr. Smith looked the other way, I turned the cuff of the jacket over, trying to sneak a peek at the price tag. I saw more zeros than I had ever seen on piece of clothing in my life. Mr. Smith caught me peeking at the price tag and quickly said, "Oh, that suit looks very nice. It's a Hickey-Freeman; it never goes on sale."

Well, the suit did look nice and suddenly I heard myself saying something I couldn't believe: "I'll take it!" (I think maybe I was shamed into buying it). Immediately a tailor came out and began to mark me up to make sure the suit fit perfectly. In the course of measuring the jacket he said, "Did you know that you have one arm longer than the other?" I am over 50 years old and I must admit I did not know that one arm was longer than the other. I couldn't wait until this guy measured my inseam!

The tailor said, "Don't worry, we'll put a shoulder pad on one side and this coat will look spiffy." I've gone from looking like a clown at Britches to looking spiffy at Nordstrom—well worth the zeros.

Nearly a week later I came back to pick up my spiffy Hickey-Freeman suit, and as luck would have it, Mr. Smith was there, as was the same tailor. It was actually the night before we were to give one of our customer service talks and I was excited about getting this new suit. Mr. Smith said, "Just take a few minutes to try it on to make sure it fits." I thought, "I'm sure it's fine, there's no need to try it on." But Mr. Smith was insistent—such is the customer service at Nordstrom. I went back into the changing room and put the pants on. Unbelievably, these pants were cut so short that you could see at least four inches of my bare legs above my socks. I shook my head, thinking, "This can't be happening. These must be someone else's pants!" I walked out of the changing room wearing the pants and Mr. Smith looked at me and said, "Put on the coat." I looked at him with fire in my eyes said, "There's no *need* to put on the coat. Look at these pants!"

"Don't worry," he said, "We'll fix the pants. Just put on the coat to see how it fits."

I gave the pants to the tailor, put on my own, and walked out wearing the coat. Looking in the mirror, I realized that the collar was puckered along the entire length of my neck. I turned to the tailor and said, "What is wrong with the collar?"

He said, "It needs pressing."

"If it needed pressing, why didn't you *press* it?" I said.

I then proceeded to cool my heels by gentlemen's ties, while they hurriedly "whittled" on my pants and pressed my coat. The tailor returned in a few minutes and flipped the coat to me like I was some sort of growth on his backside and said, "See if this isn't better." Putting on the coat, I looked at myself in the three-way mirror with the nice bright Nordstrom lights above me and realized that indeed, the collar was now smooth. However, both lapels were now so rippled that they looked like waterfalls on the front of my coat. Another salesman happened to pass by as Mr. Smith was busy with another customer, and I asked him, "What do you think is wrong with this jacket?"

He took one quick glance and said, "Oh, that is flawed. That should have never gotten by the Hickey-Freeman inspectors." Well, I know where the flaw was, and it wasn't at Hickey-Freeman. It was with Moe and Curly in the back.

I quickly changed into my clothes, found Mr. Smith and said, "I am out of here. Keep the suit and give me a refund." He did so, somewhat reluctantly, and as I was walking out of the door, he said, "Please come back—and next time I'll make sure you see our *good* tailor." Do you think that helped? Of course not, it made it worse. Effectively saying "We can't get good help" *never* makes it better.

What's the point? Nordstrom may be one of the customer service retail leaders—and it is. Betsy Sanders may be evangelical and eloquent about customer service—and she is. Her book may be so good that we bought it by the case and gave it away—and we did. But for me, Nordstrom will forever be that tailor, that salesman, and that suit. It is 100 percent of my experience with Nordstrom. My moment of truth represented service failure, not service excellence. As we said at the outset, *from the customers' perspective, the people performing the service are the company.*

Nordstrom is a service excellence leader in American retailing precisely because this story is the exception, not the rule. No one knows this better than Nordstrom itself. All of this leads us to the critical importance of the people providing the service in healthcare and the concept that *service excellence must be earned with every encounter, every day, 24/7/365.*

Some examples of the implications of the moments of truth follow:

- Fly the service excellence flag: Make service rounds on the patient care units; make it a protected part of each week (each *day* is better); put it on your schedule—make it inviolate, nothing can make you cancel it.

- Insist on your department directors and unit managers following the same policy: Leaders lead in service by being service champions.
- Ask yourself next time you are in a meeting, "Is this more important than service rounds?"
- Have nursing directors greet each new patient personally, including scripts (see below): "Please let me know if I can help you." This creates a positive expectation, whereas "Please let me know if you have any problems" creates a negative expectation.
- Use business cards liberally: Each nurse, physician, physician assistant, and nurse practitioner at BestPractices hospitals has a card with their title and name (the nurses have last initial only, for privacy purposes). They hand these to patients and families, saying, "It's been my pleasure to serve you—please contact me if I can be of help."
- Ask patients and families, "What can we do to improve our service?"
  1. "How could we do this better?"
  2. "What needs do you have that we haven't met?"
- Tell patients, "I know you have choices in healthcare. We're delighted you chose our hospital."

These are only a few of the hundreds of ways moments of truth can be enacted in your healthcare system.

MOMENTS OF TRUTH—HIRE RIGHT

Both Carlzon's concept of *Moments of Truth* and the Nordstrom story make clear the following: *The hiring of a new employee may be the most expensive decision you ever make.*

We believe that you must hire for customer service—that you must screen for the customer service gene. How true is that belief in the hiring practices in your hospital? Is customer service a part of the interview process? Most of us say "Yes," but there is usually a disconnect between our words and our actions. Is a customer service evaluation necessary to be hired at your facility? Are the following questions asked of potential employees?

- Have you ever had a patient who was really angry? How did you deal with that?
- When you have patients with unreasonable expectations, what do you say to them?
- How do you handle patients who complain to you?
- If one of your direct reports tells you she has "had it with all the complainers," what advice do you give her?
- Tell me about a time you felt really great about the service you provided to a patient.

If we are going to screen for the customer service gene, we need to change the questions we are asking when we interview people. Two of the best ones are:

1. What is the worst thing I'm going to hear about you?
2. Who am I going to hear it from?

You can also ask their previous supervisor:

- How does the person make other people feel?
- When you see this person's name on the schedule, how does your staff react? With smiles? Or do they poke their eyes out and run the other direction?

In fact, the central focus of hiring right is to *check the qualities as closely as you check the qualifications.*

When you hire staff, you check with their colleges, but do you check with their colleagues? The curriculum vitae will tell you if they received honors, but do they have honor? Their education is

Hire Right	
Qualifications	**Qualities**
• Employer	• Employees
• College(s)	• Colleagues
• Honors	• Honor
• Education	• Ethics
• Aptitude	• Attitude
• Degree(s)	• Demeanor
• Credentials	• Credibility
• Intelligence	• Integrity
• Computer skills	• Customer skills

apparent for all to see, but what about their ethics? Their transcripts and job evaluations can tell you about their intelligence, but shouldn't you also ask about their integrity? Hiring right requires that you pay attention to *both* columns. Think about this—if you had to change the attributes in one column versus the other, which would be easier to change? Without question, the attributes in the "Qualities" column are far more difficult, perhaps impossible, to change. You can train people, you can send them back to school, you can give them technical skills, and you can improve their qualifications. But if you have a "qualities loser" you most likely have a loser for life. Regardless of how tough hiring is, regardless of the shortage of workers, stay away from qualities losers. Why? *It only takes one B-team member to destroy an entire shift.* The effect that hiring a loser in the right-hand column has on morale is devastating. At BestPractices, Inc., our physician application requires that each applicant list three patients and three nurses we can call as customer service references.

Equally as important is the effect that your hiring decision will have on future hiring decisions; *First-rate people hire first-rate people. Second-rate people hire third-rate people.* First-rate people always seek to surround themselves with excellence. They know that truly great leaders hire people who can possibly even outperform them in a given area. But the team is made stronger for these skills, especially when those skills are superior. That is how an organization improves.

Second-rate people, on the other hand, always feel in competition with their own team members, in part because of their fundamental feelings of inadequacy. So instead of hiring someone at their own perceived level of competence, they hire someone *below* that level—a third-rate person—who will not challenge them. This is a doubly bankrupt strategy: Not only are they hiring down but their own feelings of inadequacy cause them to underestimate their own true potential.

THE OPEN BOOK TEST APPROACH TO PATIENT SATISFACTION SURVEYS

Measuring or reporting on patient satisfaction has become a central focus for healthcare institutions. Indeed, it has become an important industry unto itself. Virtually every healthcare system measures patient satisfaction with inpatient and outpatient services and reports these results to the board. Satisfaction matters, no question about it. However, much of the failure to improve patient satisfaction rests with this issue: *Are your surveys a tool, or a club?*

In other words, are the scores used as a tool to help you to improve your services, your process, and your employee's skills? Or are the scores used as a club to bludgeon staff with threats and imprecations? Are your department managers saying, "Get those scores up or…"? Or what? "We'll fire them?" With current staffing shortages? "We'll make them worker harder, longer, for less money?" You get the point—start with a fundamental understanding that measuring patient satisfaction should be used as a tool to help make the job easier, not as a punitive measure.

An equally important insight regarding patient satisfaction surveys is best illustrated from a story of one of our sons. Josh (now a graduate of Dartmouth College) came home from school one day during his eighth grade year with a demeanor that could only mean he had a bad day. The following father-son conversation occurred:

Dad: Josh, you look like you had a bad day. What happened?
Josh: I had a test and I flunked it.
Dad: Josh, did you know you were going to have this test?
Josh: Of course I did.

As those of you with children know, there are a couple of additional questions a parent is compelled to ask.

Dad: Josh, this test that you knew you were going to have and that
      you are certain you failed, what sort of test was it?
Josh: It was an open book test, Dad.
Dad (somewhat stunned): Did you happen to *open the book*, Josh?
Josh: No, Dad. I didn't even take the book to school.

Somehow I resisted the overriding urge to ask the only logical follow-up question: "Josh, was the term 'moron' on this test? 'Imbecile?' You had an open book test and you didn't even open the book?"

You get the point: *Your patient satisfaction survey is an open book test.*

All of us know—or could choose to know—the questions on the test before they are asked. Does your staff know what the questions are on your patient satisfaction survey? If not, they're like Josh— the book is right there, waiting to be opened, but they choose not to open it. Use the open book test approach to patient satisfaction surveys.

- Review the questions proactively with the staff.
- Huddle up with the staff and discuss appropriate A-team behaviors for each of the questions on the test.
- Use scripts to encourage these A-team behaviors.

- Search for and eliminate the B-team behaviors that might occur.
- Empower the staff to find ways to use the open book test approach where the survey is a tool, not a club.

Most surveys have questions for doctors, nurses, laboratory, radiology, etc. It's a generally good idea to have each of these segments review these questions themselves and come up with their own A-team behaviors and scripts. However, it is also a good idea to circulate those responses between areas of the team, so that nurses review doctors' questions, doctors review nurses' questions, etc. This is truly a team approach to the open book test.

DESIGNING A-TEAM BEHAVIORS AND SCRIPTS

Brainstorm during staff meetings and discuss the A-team behaviors and scripts openly—the solution should be theirs, not yours. To be sure, there is a role for senior leadership as a catalyst in the open book test approach, but the actual scripts themselves are better designed by those who will use them.

After the scripts have been developed for each area, exchange them so team members can comment and further develop each other's areas. This is a true test of team behavior—the ability to candidly, but with sensitivity, comment on the A-team and B-team behaviors of the other team members.

MOMENTS OF TRUTH—SCRIPTS

We emphasize the importance of understanding that your patient satisfaction surveys are an open book test. Moreover, the A-team behaviors and B-team behaviors, when discussed openly with your staff, are truly obvious to all. Since this is the case, why not use pre-determined scripts, designed by your A-team members, to help guide your staff through predictable, frequent, and even problem-prone areas in healthcare? In fact, your staff are already doing the hard work of providing technical and clinical care—the A-team behaviors. Why not design scripts that help alert the patient, their family, and the other team members in healthcare that they are doing a good job? Scripts can be extremely helpful in this regard by emphasizing to the patient and their family the work that is actually being done—the A-team behaviors being exhibited every day.

Many effective scripts fall into the category of *previews*. Previews in healthcare are similar to previews in a movie theater—they give us a glimpse of what is coming, the "future attractions." Scripts should be focused, specific, and designed to help guide patient expectations, as we emphasized in Chapter 4. The following are effective preview scripts:

- "The chest x ray will take about 45 minutes."
- "We typically expect you to be in the hospital for five days following a hip replacement. Each day, the nurses and I will let you know how you are doing as you proceed through your journey."
- "Since you've tolerated the angioplasty extremely well, I expect that we will transfer you out to the telemetry unit later this evening."

One of the most powerful scripts for patients in any area of healthcare is, "Do you have any questions? I have plenty of time." Patients are going to have questions. Family members are going to have questions. Aunt Edna who just flew in from Oklahoma is going to have *a lot* of questions. Let the patients know that you expect to answer their questions. Give them note pads to write these questions down so they can remember them. Some of your staff will tell you that they don't have time for all of these questions. However, this isn't really spending time; it's investing time, by proactively letting the patient and their family know that you will answer all of their questions. They are going to come anyway; you might as well get them up front. Some of the more powerful scripts are:

- "I'm Bill Smith, the hospital CEO. How can we improve the way we do things here?"
- "I'm sorry this happened to you."
- "I'm Dr. Evans, the cardiologist. Your personal physician asked me to come by and visit with you. I've read the nurses' notes and I understand that...."
- "Randy is one of our best nurses—you are fortunate to have him taking care of you today."
- "I'm Nancy Lopez, the patient care director on this unit. I just wanted to stop by and make sure you knew who I was and that service is very important to us. Please let us know if there is anything we can do for you."
- "Making sure you are comfortable is important to us. The IV fluids and the medications we've given you should help with that, but let us know if you aren't feeling better in the next 25 to 30 minutes."
- "Mrs. Scott, I'm Candace Bell, the chief operating officer of the hospital. I understand there was a problem with your service. I'm sorry that happened. How can I be of help?"
- "Mrs. Jones, I'll be your nurse on 4 East. We've been expecting you! I've talked with your nurse in the emergency department, so I feel I already know you. I'm looking forward to taking care of you."

The list is truly endless, because the number of A-team behaviors in your institution is endless. Scripting simply empowers your staff to use these A-team behaviors and turn them into scripts that can be shared with their colleagues. These will create phenomenal moments of truth as success breeds success and A-team behaviors generate even more A-team behaviors.

MOMENTS OF TRUTH—TEAMWORK

Throughout healthcare, the importance of teamwork is emphasized. If you ask anyone in healthcare if they are a team, they will invariably answer, "Oh, yes. Team, team, team. See the poster on the wall that says we are?" Of course, posters and slogans do not make a team. We believe you can spend an hour on any healthcare unit in the country and tell by the interactions between the people whether they operate as a team or not. Teamwork is one of the fundamental pieces of success in healthcare customer service. *The #1 reason to get customer service right is that it makes the job easier through A-team behaviors and A-team attitudes.* The A-team makes work easier.

We recently had the honor and privilege of spending a weekend aboard the nuclear aircraft carrier USS George Washington, which was a truly transforming experience. Among many lessons learned from observing these men and women in uniform, the most important is their dedication and commitment to teamwork. The 4.5 acres comprising the flight deck of a nuclear aircraft carrier is the most dangerous territory on earth. Fighter and attack jets, fully armed with ordnance, are catapulted off a deck splashed with oil and seawater, accelerating from a standstill to 150 miles per hour in less than 2 seconds by catapults with 2 million horsepower. Aircraft are recovered in cycles at the opposite end of the flight deck by other members of the team, each with specific duties. The roar is deafening, even with earplugs and protective headgear, so communications among the team are accomplished by an elaborate yet widely understood set of hand signals. Each step of the choreography interrelates closely with the others, from raising the aircraft off the hanger deck via elevators to the flight deck, through positioning the aircraft in an elegant series of moves to the catapult, through their explosive launch. The flight deck crew wear brightly colored shirts, each color designating their role on the team, including red for ordnance (the folks who load the bombs and missiles), white for safety officers, green for catapult and recovery wire operators, yellow for launch personnel (the "shooters"), and silver flame-proof suits for the elite fire and recovery team. While the lessons learned from observing carrier operations would fill an entire book, their teamwork is clearly something all of us in healthcare can aspire toward. We asked to see the training manuals describing the elaborate ballet of personnel and machinery. Somewhat sheepishly the captain replied, "We don't have one; these procedures are passed down verbally—and accurately—among our crew."

How can we communicate the importance of teamwork in our training? Here's a story we first heard from legendary football coach Lou Holtz.

I was scheduled to give a talk not far from Charlotte, North Carolina, one night, but as luck would have it, my plane arrived late on this rainy evening. I dashed off in the rental car and drove further and further into the hills of North Carolina on the rain-soaked roads.

Fortunately, the rain stopped, but I was still running late, and as I looked over to check the map, I slid off the road into a ditch, where my rental car was mired helplessly in the mud. But today was my lucky day! A farmer emerged out of the mist on the road, and he was leading a huge, old plow horse he called Buddy. I waved the farmer down and asked if he could help me. The old fellow looked at me, looked at my car, and looked back at Buddy—and then he said, "Yep, I believe I can help you. You get in the car, put it into neutral, and steer."

He pulled out a rope and tied it to the front bumper of my car, looped it around Buddy's harness, and tied it tightly. Cupping his hands around his mouth, he yelled, "Pull, Nellie, Pull!" Nothing happened.

Then he yelled, "Pull, Rosie, Pull!" Nothing happened.

Then he yelled, "Pull, Buster, Pull!" Nothing happened.

Then, softly, he said, "Pull, Buddy, pull."

That old horse pulled my car out of the ditch in nothing flat. My car was sitting high and dry, and I was ready to get on the road and make it to my speech. As the farmer was untying the rope from under the car and around Buddy's harness, I couldn't help but ask him, "Sir, it's none of my business, but I just noticed that you called your horse by the wrong name three times. What gives?"

The old farmer looked at me and said, "Well, you see old Buddy is blind. And if he thought he was the only one pulling, he wouldn't even try."

It's good to have a team, but sometimes we just have to get our old, blind Buddy pulling in the right direction.

REWARD YOUR CHAMPIONS

One of the best ways to ensure that your staff members feel like heroes is to tell them—and tell them and tell them. You cannot praise them enough. Celebrate their successes visibly and meaningfully. Send them notes (handwritten whenever possible) when you receive copies of compliment letters.

Betsy,
I had a chance to see the wonderful note from Mrs. Smith— a great example of your A-team attitude. Thanks so much for your help in making our hospital the nation's service excellence leader!

Many thanks,

Steve
CEO
Central Medical Center

Celebrate their successes with service legend stories and management/leadership team meetings. Read the letters from patients;

better yet, ask the patients to attend the meeting, have them tell the story, and have them present the service award.

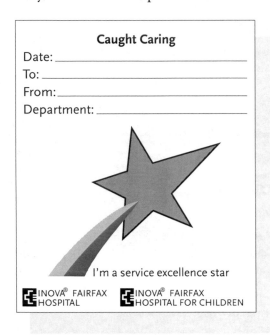

Find ways to let patients and other staff help celebrate the service excellence they see. At Inova Health System, we use the "caught caring" approach, consisting of readily available notes with adhesive backs, so patients and staff can express their appreciation. Notice the star logo on the form. Barrow Neurologic Institute /St. Joseph's Hospital in Phoenix uses a similar program with a different format.

In our emergency department, we created the Star of the ER award in an attempt to reward our champions. Each month, the employee with the best customer service ratings is given the Star (as in Starfish) of the ER award, including a plaque with his or her name and the Starfish symbol on it, as well as gift certificates totaling $200. Each quarter, a Star of the Quarter is named, who receives a MasterCard worth $500; suite tickets to the local professional hockey, football, or basketball teams (depending on the season); as well as two free first-class airline tickets (donated from the hundreds of thousands of miles we travel each year teaching customer service courses). Does this cost money? Of course. Does it pay dividends in terms of employee satisfaction? You bet. It is a very small price to pay for letting our staff know how deeply they are appreciated.

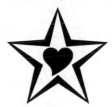

H.E.A.R.T./S.T.A.R.

- ♥ Hear the complaint
- ♥ Empathize and evaluate
- ♥ Apologize
- ♥ Resolve with urgency
- ♥ Thank the patient/
  family member

☆ Service
☆ Teamwork
☆ Accountability
☆ Respect

Person nominated: _____

Core behavior exhibited: _____

☐Hear the complaint ☐Empathize ☐Apologize ☐Resolve with urgency ☐Thank you
☐Service ☐Teamwork ☐Accountability ☐Respect

In financial terms, rewarding your champion has the best return on investment of any program in your healthcare system. These programs create employee satisfaction, service excellence legends, excitement about their jobs, and better staff retention.

- Celebrate success publicly.
- Praise liberally—and often.
- Create service legends at management meetings.
- Develop a Star of the Month/Quarter program.
- Have lunch with your award winners—hear *their* perspective.

MOMENTS OF TRUTH—THE STAR THROWER

You and your staff are involved in one of the greatest endeavors one could hope for—delivering healthcare to those in need. It is an honored and honorable calling, and each of us has a piece of the teamwork of delivering that care. It is essential that your staff understand how deeply you honor what they do. But how do you communicate that? There are many ways, but we have found the following story to be one of the most effective. It is, on its surface, a hokey story, appealing to the deepest emotions and brightest lights of your staff. For that reason, it requires a certain amount of personal courage to tell—after all, all of us are a little concerned that people will laugh and jeer, at least on the inside, at such emotional stories. However, it is a highly effective one, in our experience and that of others. It is adapted from a wonderful and incisive essay, "The Star Thrower," by the scientist Dr. Loren Eiseley. Here's how we tell it.

I should warn you at the outset that the following story is probably apocryphal and certainly sentimental, if not outright "hokey." But it's good enough that I'll risk telling it to you anyway.

In our area near Washington, D.C., many people need to take vacations for rest and relaxation. A lot of them go to the Outer Banks, the barrier islands in North Carolina, which are several hours drive away. The story is told that a businessman from our nation's capital decided to take his family, rent a house at the Outer Banks, and unwind at the beach. He checked in on a Saturday afternoon and settled his family in. As it turns out, that Saturday night there was a huge storm that howled in off of the Atlantic. The storm created a significant tidal surge, such that water came up and underneath the house he was renting. But as you may know, these houses are built on stilts so the tide simply washed up under the house and then back out to sea.

But a curious thing happened during that tidal surge. It carried so many starfish with it that, when the businessman walked out of his rented house on Sunday morning, it appeared that every starfish in the sea had been deposited on the beaches of the Outer Banks. Truly, it appeared that the sky had "rained starfish." It was early in the morning and the man looked to his left and looked to his right prior to walking down the beach. In the distance off to his left he saw someone on the beach, so he walked in that direction. As he did so, he became curious, as the figure on the beach repeatedly bent over and then stood back up, bent over and then stood back up, over and over. As he walked further in that direction, he became even more curious, because he realized it was a little girl, about nine years old. She was picking up starfish, one by one, cleaning them off, and throwing them back into the ocean.

As he reached the young girl, the businessman said, "Little girl, I couldn't help notice what you were doing as I walked toward you. I'm sorry to tell you this, but what you're doing can't possibly make any difference. I have been watching you for the last 15 minutes as I walked along," he said, "and you've only been able to clear this one small little area about seven feet around."

He continued, "There are thousands of starfish on this beach and maybe millions more that we can't even see," he said, sweeping his arm back to the right. "So, I'm sorry to tell you this, but what you're doing can't possibly make any difference."

Looking down at the starfish in her hand, the little girl said, "It does to *this* one!" as she threw the starfish back into the sea.

Well, as I said, it's a hokey story and I'm not sure it even happened.

But that's what *you* do—isn't it? Every time you take care of a patient, every time you come to work, every time you help out one of your colleagues...you make a difference in people's lives.

If you have children, ask them what they want to *do* with their lives, and they'll tell you the same thing that our children tell us—"I want to make a difference in people's lives!" There is a word for people who work hard for others, who strive valiantly, sometimes against what seems like impossible odds—and all for the good of others. Do you know what the word is? It's "hero." Here's our question to you—when you work here at our hospital and healthcare system, do you feel like a hero? You should! Because if you're not a hero, who is? You take care of those who can't, won't, or don't understand how to take care of themselves. You do it person by person, day by day, week by week, year in and year out. You do it with style, grace, dignity, and equanimity. You are a hero. You are a star thrower!

As promised, this is a hokey story—and you may think it a risky story to tell. But from extensive experience, we can assure you that it is a highly effective story. In many respects, the sum of the message of moments of truth is contained within that story. We have told it to thousands of people at hundreds of hospitals, all with dramatic effect. We invite you to do the same. At our institution, all of our new hires hear the star thrower story. Appropriately enough, our employees of the month and of the quarter are known as the Stars of the ER. They receive, along with their gift certificates and credit cards, a framed certificate with a logo—a starfish.

Whether you use this story or another, it's important that you find a way to help your staff understand that they not only make a difference in people's lives but they are also heroes. This is the essence of any successful service excellence program—helping the A-team understand that, not only is their hard work deeply appreciated (reward your champions) but it is truly heroic work—playing a part in serving others in the time of their deepest need, when their health or that of their family and loved ones is at stake. Our fondest hope is that these three Survival Skills

1. Making the customer service diagnosis as well as the technical diagnosis and offering the right treatment
2. Negotiating for agreement and resolution expectations
3. Creating moments of truth

will combine to achieve two fundamental goals for you and your staff:

- Goal #1—To make the job easier (the real reason to develop service excellence)
- Goal #2—To help you and your staff realize anew that you are engaged in one of the world's most honored professions—giving care and comfort to those who entrust their lives and health to us.

In closing, we turn to the words of a truly great human being, Albert Schweitzer, M.D. (1998):

Of all the will toward the ideal in mankind, only a small part can manifest itself in public action. All the rest of this force must be content with small and obscure deeds. The sum of these, however, is a thousand times stronger than the acts of those who receive wild public recognition. The latter, compared to the former, are like the foam on the waves of a deep ocean.

We gain great satisfaction from teaching service excellence to our colleagues in healthcare across this great nation. But as we travel and come to know people like you and your staff, we realize how true Dr. Schweitzer's words are—we are like the foam on the deep ocean of the good works that you and your staff do. Our hope is that our work makes your work a little easier.

SURVIVAL SKILLS SUMMARY

- Your staff constantly creates moments of truth for patients thousands of times a day—the sum of which create the reputation of your healthcare system.
- The third Survival Skill is *creating moments of truth*.
- From the customer's perspective, the people performing the service *are* the company.
- Better to have one person practicing empowered customer service than a hundred posted mission statements proclaiming it.
- It's not the mission statement, it's your staff in action that creates service in the organization.
- Service excellence is never complete—it has to be earned every day, in every patient encounter.
- As the leader, round regularly and visibly on the patient units.
- Solve service problems—on the spot.
- Patient care unit directors should greet every admitted patient and give them their card, a smile, and the reassurance that "I'm here to help if you need me."

- Hire right—screen for the customer service gene.
- Hiring a new employee is the most expensive decision you will make.
- Make customer service a meaningful and decisive part of the interview process.
- Check the qualities as closely as you check the qualifications.
- Don't forget that first-rate people hire first-rate people, but second-rate people hire third-rate people.
- Use your surveys as a tool, not a club.
- Patient satisfaction surveys are an open book test.
- Use the open book test approach—huddle up.
  —Analyze each question for A-team and B-team behaviors.
  —Recognize the power of scripts.
  —Develop scripts to accentuate A-team behaviors—service excellence.
- Provide ongoing feedback, using the surveys as an open book, as well as complaint and compliment analysis.
- Reward your champions.
- Celebrate success—create service legends.
- Tell the star thrower story to help your staff understand that what they do is fundamentally heroic—and they are heros!

REFERENCES

Eiseley, L. 1978. "The Star Thrower." In *The Star Thrower*, 169–85. Fort Washington, PA: Harvest Books.

Schweitzer, A. 1998. *Out of My Life and Work*. Baltimore, MD: John Hopkins University Press.

MORE ON THIS

Block, P. 2002. *The Answer to How is Yes*. San Francisco: Berrett-Koehler.
A truly inspirational book from one of the most incisive minds writing about leadership.

Carlzon, J. 1987. *Moments of Truth: New Strategies for Today's Customer-Driven Economy.* New York: Harper Collins.
The book that defined and launched the concept of moments of truth, with an insightful forward by Tom Peters.

Greenleaf, R. K. 2002. *Servant Leadership: A Journey into the Nature of Legitimate Power and Greatness.* New York: Paulist Press.
A collection of essays defining servant leadership, including Greenleaf's seminal essay launching the concept of servant leadership. Essays by Stephen Covey and Peter Senge are also excellent.

Kotter, J. P. 1996. *Leading Change.* Boston: Harvard Business School Press.
The definitive text on change management, an essential tool for any service excellence initiative.

Press, I. 2002. *Patient Satisfaction: Defining, Measuring, and Improving the Experience of Care.* Chicago: Health Administration Press.
A scholarly and detailed approach from the nation's éminence grise in patient satisfaction surveys—and a great friend.

Sanders. B. 1995. *Fabled Service: Ordinary Acts, Extraordinary Outcomes.* San Diego: Pfieffer.
A fast but good read, blending elements of the Nordstrom philosophy with great insights and quotes from Tom Peters, Sum Wattson, Jan Carlzon, and Mother Theresa.

Two brief books with insights from two service industry leaders.

Spector, R., and P. McCarthy. 1995. *The Nordstrom Way.* New York: John Wiley.

Connellan, T. 1997. *Inside the Magic Kingdom: Seven Keys to Disney's Success.* Austin, TX: Bard Press.

Putting Survival Skills to Work

HOW DO YOU apply the Survival Skills concept to your institution? Consider this last section a "how to" manual, designed to turn it over to the troops to implement. If you and your staff understand and apply these concepts, your service excellence will succeed, with one very critical caveat: *This journey is never over; there is no finish line; and success occurs one action at a time, one patient at a time, every hour of every day of every year.*

GETTING STARTED

- Healthcare is a personal service business—the unit of measure is one person caring for another person.
- Most service initiatives are presented as one more task, one more initiative among many—that's why they fail.
- Help your staff understand that the #1 reason to adopt a customer service initiative is *it makes the job easier.*
- A-team behaviors make the job easier and create patient compliments.

- B-team behaviors make the job harder and create patient complaints.
- It only takes one B-team member to destroy an entire shift.

FOCUS ON A-TEAM BEHAVIORS—THEY MAKE THE JOB EASIER

- Use compliment analysis to identify A-team behaviors and spread them throughout the organization.
- Use the A-team/B-team exercise to show the staff they're already involved in providing good customer service—they just haven't called it that or demanded it from everyone.
- Show your staff it's as easy as 1–2–3:
  1. Make clear there's a fundamental, universal, and lasting cultural change toward service excellence.
  2. Hire right, train right, promote right, and create a service vocabulary for your staff.
  3. Make it a part of the daily experience—and shoot the stragglers.
- Use the "Are they patients or customers?" exercise to demonstrate that we subconsciously classify those we care for by this simple diagnostic rule: The more horizontal they are, the more they're a patient. The more vertical they are, the more they're a customer.
- Show them that the % patient added to the % customer always equals 100%. Treat the % patient with technical skills and the % customer with service skills.
- Demonstrate the first Survival Skill—*making the customer service diagnosis and offering the right treatment*—by
  —Anticipating experiences from the customer/patient's viewpoint
  —Building your healthcare processes around the patient's viewpoint

—Using expectation creation—let the patient and family know what to expect and act as their guide through healthcare
—Developing and sharing scripts to accentuate A-team behaviors
- Demonstrate the second Survival Skill—*negotiating agreement and resolution of expectations*—by teaching the three negotiation steps and the six negotiation tools:

Negotiation Steps
1. Discovering your expectations
2. Discovering their expectations
3. Negotiating expectations for inventing options for mutual gain

Negotiation Tools
1. Empowerment
2. Point-of-impact intervention
3. Service recovery
4. Dealing with difficult patients
5. Dealing with B-team members
6. Dealing with B-team bosses

- Demonstrate the third Survival Skill—*building moments of truth into the healthcare encounter*—by showing them that
—From the customer's viewpoint, the people performing the service are the company
—It is better to have one employee practicing empowered customer service than to have 100 posted vision statements proclaiming it
—Frequent service rounds on patient care units are invaluable
—Scripting for moments of truth spread service quickly—use them again and again
—Patient satisfaction surveys are an open book test—huddle up and discuss the questions and scripts for A-team behaviors
—You seek out and celebrate your service champions

—You reward your champions

—You help your staff understand that what they do is fundamentally heroic by using the star thrower story (or another of your choosing)

ELIMINATE B-TEAM BEHAVIORS—THEY DESTROY MORALE

- Use complaint analysis to identify and eliminate B-team behaviors.
- Make sure your staff understands there's a new sheriff in town—one who won't let Dr. Torquemada, Nurse Ratched, or Administrator Scrooge run wild anymore.
- Hire right—screen for the customer service gene.
- Check the *qualities* as closely as you check the *qualifications*.
- Don't take a short-term solution (a B-team member) to a long-term problem (sustaining service excellence in your organization)—no matter how bad staffing might be.
- Don't forget that *hiring an employee is the most expensive decision you'll ever make.*
- Remember that *first-rate people hire first-rate people, but second-rate people hire third-rate people.*
- Learn to deal with B-team members—be clear, be specific, show concern, let them know how their behavior affects others (When you do *x*, it makes others feel *y*), give them an example of an A-team behavior ("Try *z*"), and tie it all back to the service excellence strategy.
- Give B-team members the remedial course. If they fail that, don't be afraid to…
- Fire right; if Dr. Torquemada, Nurse Ratched, or Administrator Scrooge can't get with the program, they need to get gone.

SUSTAINING SUCCESS

- Make service excellence a central part of every staff meeting at every level of the organization.
- Continue compliment and complaint analysis to accelerate A-team behavior and circumscribe—and then eliminate—B-team behaviors.
- Don't just say "team"—*live* teamwork.
- Service rounds on patient care units are essential; sadly, many CEOs are never seen down in the trenches.
- Celebrate service success—bring patients and families to leadership team meetings to recognize the Star of the Month, service legends, or whatever you choose to call them.
- Reward your champions, whether with praise, recognition, cash, parking spaces, or tickets to events (better yet, ask them what *they* want and give it to them).

Is it really that simple? *Can* it be that simple? Frankly, *yes*. Don't focus on scores or market share. Focus on making your staff's job easier. Focus on A-team and B-team behaviors your staff will understand because they live this every day at work. Create a vocabulary of service, a taxonomy, a way of describing Stars of the Month—or whatever you decide to call them. Celebrate successes and reward your champions. Service excellence is all around us—the problem is that we are inconsistent at it. We've traditionally described customer service in ways that make it sound like one more thing we're tasking our staff with. It needs to be presented so they understand that customer service—A-team behaviors and attitudes—make their jobs easier.

Help your staff understand that we are involved in one of the greatest, most timeless, most honorable professions in the entire world—caring for, curing of, and comforting those who need our help. Good luck with this. For those whose deep joy arises from meeting the deep needs of others, it is the most honorable and fulfilling work on the earth.

Suggested Readings

Argyris, C. 1993. *Knowledge for Action: A Guide to Overcoming Barriers to Organizational Change*. San Francisco: Jossey-Bass.
One the finest sources on organizational change, including insights on the importance of the difference between espoused and enacted strategies.

Belasco, J. A., and R. C. Stayer. 1993. *The Flight of the Buffalo*. New York: Warner Books.

Berry, L. L. 1999. *Discovering the Soul of Service: The Nine Drivers of Sustainable Business Success*. New York: The Free Press.
Len Berry is the preeminent source concerning the science of service. This study of 14 service industry leaders has many lessons for healthcare.

Berry, L. L., and N. Bendapudi. 2003. "Clueing in Customers." *Harvard Business Review* 81 (2): 100–106.
Service from the customer's perspective at the Mayo Clinic, as seen through the eyes of a legend in service writings.

Each of these books is excellent and contains good sections on service recovery.

Block, P. 2002. *The Right Use of Power: How Stewardship Replaces Leadership*. Louisville, CO: Sounds True.
Audio/CD available at PeterBlock.com.
Peter Block, in his own voice, with penetrating analysis for leaders at all levels.

———. 2002. *The Answer to How is Yes*. San Francisco: Berrett-Koehler.
A truly inspirational book from one of the most incisive minds writing about leadership.

Nearly every page of our copy is dog-eared, is heavily underlined, or has notes written in the margin.

Bossidy, L., and R. Charn. 2002. *Execution: The Discipline of Getting Things Done*. New York: Crown Business.
A terrific book that explains why it is easy to have a great idea but difficult to execute the idea in practice.

Carlzon, J. 1987. *Moments of Truth: New Strategies for Today's Customer-Driven Economy*. New York: Harper Collins.
The book that defined and launched the concept of moments of truth, with an insightful foreword by Tom Peters.

Connellan, T. 1997. *Inside the Magic Kingdom: Seven Keys to Disney's Success*. Austin, TX: Bard Press.
Insights from a service industry leader.

Fisher, R., W. Ury, and B. Patton. 1991. *Getting to Yes: Negotiating Agreement Without Giving In*, 2nd ed. New York: Penguin.

Ury, W. 1993. *Getting Past No: Negotiating Your Way From Confrontation to Cooperation*. New York: Bantam.

———. 1999. *Getting to Peace: Transforming Conflict at Home, at Work, and in the World*. New York: Penguin.

The best of the books on negotiation, all of which are very practical. The first book is an essential read on negotiation.

Frieberg, K., and J. Frieberg. 1997. *Nuts! Southwest Airlines' Crazy Recipe for Business and Personal Success*. New York: Broadway Books.

Gitomer, J. 1998. *Customer Satisfaction is Worthless: Customer Loyalty is Priceless*. Austin, TX: Bard Press.

Gladwell, M. 2002. *The Tipping Point: How Little Things Can Make a Big Difference*. San Francisco: Back Bay Books.
A brief but helpful book showing how inflection points can make all the difference in change management.

Greenleaf, R. K. 2002. *Servant Leadership: A Journey into the Nature of Legitimate Power and Greatness*. New York: Paulist Press.
A collection of essays defining servant leadership, including Greenleaf's seminal essay launching the concept of servant leadership. Essays by Stephen Covey and Peter Senge are also excellent.

Kotter, J. P. 1996. *Leading Change*. Boston: Harvard Business School Press.
The definitive text on change management, an essential tool for any service excellence initiative.

Maslow, A. H. 1998. *Maslow on Management*. New York: Wiley.
An absolute treasure of insights from one of the greatest psychologists of all time, which includes a foreword by Warren Bennis.

Mayer, T. A., and R. J. Cates. 1999. "Service Excellence in Health Care." *Journal of the American Medical Association* 282 (13): 1281–83.

Mayer, T. A., R. J. Cates, M. J. Mastorovich, and D. L. Royalty. 1998. "Emergency Department Patient Satisfaction." *Journal of Healthcare Management* 43 (5): 427–40.

These short articles from both the medical and business literature range from defining patients and customers to strategies for change in healthcare. All are essential reads.

Berwick, D. M. 2003. "Disseminating Innovations in Healthcare." *Journal of the American Medical Association* 289: 1969–75.

Patterson, K., J. Grenny, R. McMillan, A. Switzler, and S. Covey. 2002. *Crucial Conversations: Tools for Talking When the the Stakes are High*. New York: McGraw-Hill.
A great book on turning dysfunctional communication into powerful connections.

Peters, T. 2003. *Re-imagine!* New York: Dorling Kindersly.
The latest from the incomparable and essential Tom Peters—a great resource and a great read from an international treasure. There are great discoveries on each page.

Press, I. 2002. *Patient Satisfaction: Defining, Measuring, and Improving the Experience of Care*. Chicago: Health Administration Press.
A scholarly and detailed approach from the nation's éminence grise in patient satisfaction surveys—and a great friend.

Sanders, B. 1995. *Fabled Service: Ordinary Acts, Extraordinary Outcomes*. San Diego: Pfieffer.
A fast but good read, blending elements of the Nordstrom philosophy with great insights and quotes from Tom Peters, Sam Walton, Jan Carlzon, and Mother Theresa.

Schweitzer, A. 1998. *Out of My Life and Work*. Baltimore, MD: Johns Hopkins University Press.
The powerful autobiography of a great physician, the importance of which has not diminished over the years.

Selye, H. 1978. *The Stress of Life*. New York: McGraw-Hill.
The seminal work on stress, which has retained its pertinence more than 50 years after its original publication.

Spector, R., and P. McCarthy. 1995. *The Nordstrom Way*. New York: John Wiley.
Insights from a retail service industry leader.

About the Authors

Thom A. Mayer, M.D., is president and chief executive officer of BestPractices, Inc., a national resource in physician leadership and management.

Dr. Mayer has been the keynote speaker at numerous healthcare leadership conferences and also serves as the medical director of the NFL Players Association. He is one of America's foremost experts on healthcare customer service, trauma and emergency care, pediatric emergency care, and medical leadership. He has published over 60 articles and 60 book chapters and has edited 10 medical textbooks.

On September 11, 2001, Dr. Mayer served as one of the command physicians at the Pentagon Rescue Operation, coordinating medical assets at the site. The BestPractices physicians at Inova Fairfax Hospital were the first to successfully diagnose and treat inhalational anthrax victims during the 2001 anthrax crises. Dr. Mayer is the lead editor of *Emergency Department Management: Principles and Applications*, the benchmark text on emergency leadership, and has served the Department of Defense on the Defense Science Board Task Forces on Bioterrorism and Homeland Security.

Robert (Bob) J. Cates, M.D., is a practicing emergency department physician and chairman of the Inova Fairfax Hospital's department of emergency medicine in Falls Church, Virginia. Under Dr. Cates's leadership, the emergency department has won numerous awards and grants, most recently the prestigious Robert Wood Johnson Foundation Urgent Matters Grant.

Dr. Cates received his undergraduate degree at Southern Illinois University, his master's degree in biochemistry at Indiana University, and his M.D. at Indiana University. His postgraduate training included a medicine internship at Indiana University Medical Center, a medicine residency at Georgetown University, and four years as a clinical associate and staff associate at the National Institutes of Health (NIH) in the Cancer Institute. He is a widely sought speaker on the application of customer service in healthcare.